A Fireside Book
Published by
Simon & Schuster
New York London
Toronto Sydney
Tokyo Singapore

THE WATERLOVER'S GUIDE

TO MARINE MEDICINE

PAUL G. GILL, JR., M.D.

FIRESIDE
SIMON & SCHUSTER BUILDING
ROCKEFELLER CENTER
1230 AVENUE OF THE AMERICAS
NEW YORK, NEW YORK 10020

DESIGNED BY PEI LOI KOAY
ILLUSTRATED BY WILLIAM P. HAMILTON
DRAWING BY PAUL G. GILL, JR., M.D. APPEARS ON PAGE 5

MANUFACTURED IN THE UNITED STATES OF AMERICA

1 3 5 7 9 10 8 6 4 2

LIBRARY OF CONGRESS CATALOGING-IN-PUBLICATION DATA
GILL, PAUL G., DATE.
THE WATERLOVER'S GUIDE TO MARINE MEDICINE / PAUL G. GILL, JR.
P. CM.
"A FIRESIDE BOOK."
INCLUDES INDEX.
1. MEDICINE, NAVAL. 2. FIRST AID IN ILLNESS AND INJURY. I. TITLE.
[DNLM: 1. FIRST AID. 2. NAVAL MEDICINE. WA 292 G475W 1993]
RC986.G55 1993
616.9'8024—DC20
DNLM/DLC
FOR LIBRARY OF CONGRESS   93-479
CIP
ISBN: 0-671-79452-3

For two Sons of Aran,

My grandfather, Captain William F. Gill, who went to

sea at the age of ten, and sailed before the mast

around Cape Horn,

and

My father, Paul G. Gill, Sr., Third Officer of the

SS Nathanael Greene during its voyages to

Archangel, U.S.S.R., and North Africa in 1942–43.

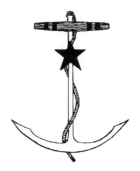

CONTENTS

•

•

•

•

FOREWORD

Dr. Paul G. Gill, Jr., and I have much in common. We are both sportsmen who have a great love for the sea. Paul's ancestors were fishermen and sailors, and he has not strayed from his heritage. I have owned boats for more than forty years, fishing the offshore waters of the East Coast every chance I get.

Like Paul, I cannot abide water that does not smell of salt, flood the marsh grass with a tide, or give me the opportunity to catch striped bass and blue crabs. I have enormous pity for people who do not understand the importance of "messin' around with boats" and the unmatchable exhilaration of running an inlet in the face of a flaming rising sun. What great adventure not to know what lies ahead for you and your boat that day! Unfortunately, what sometimes lies ahead can also be a mess of trouble.

One of the most heartbreaking incidents in my personal experience was when my two-year-old grandson Nicholas flopped down in a shallow tidal pool on a family "gunkholing" adventure and landed on a jellyfish. As soon as I saw the red blotch on his stomach, I knew why he was screaming in pain. You can sometimes explain pain away with an adult, but never with a two-year-old child. I knew about some remedies, such as a baking soda and water paste, but I did not have these things on my boat. He cried until he had no more tears that day. Now I carry jellyfish and stingray treatment kits.

Boats can give you a true sense of freedom, but they can also be very dangerous places. I have seen experienced boat people fall overboard, drive fishhooks into their fingers, get seasick, break toes, bang heads, burn skin under a searing sun, strain backs, and on and on. None of these things would probably have happened if they had stayed home and watched a ballgame. But I can't imagine giving up a day on the water for television or for anything else short of showing up to collect on a lottery ticket. Obviously, the only solution is to train yourself to handle the emergencies that are likely to happen on a boat, and I can't think of a better teacher than a doctor who has the sea in his blood.

Paul Gill started his regular sports medicine column for *Outdoor Life* back in 1988. Paul is a board-certified emergency medicine specialist and a member of the Wilderness Medical Society, but what really got him his job at *Outdoor Life* was his background as a hunter, fisherman, and camper. Paul's first book, *Simon & Schuster's Pocket Guide to Wilderness Medicine,* was a resounding success. I keep copies in my home, truck, and deer camp. While on a grouse hunt, I used it as a guide for treating a friend's scratched cornea.

Paul's new book, *The Waterlover's Guide to Marine Medicine,* is a natural companion to that first volume. You will find twenty chapters in this book, ranging from shipboard dentistry to seasickness to fish poisoning to whatever else could occur while fishing or cruising. Did you know, for example, that stewed tomatoes or Chinese apples may cure your seasickness? Or that you can get double vision by picking up cone shells in shallow water?

Paul covers a great variety of emergencies and ailments in his treatment of marine medicine. His writing is short, clear, and crisp . . . in itself a major accomplishment for a medical doctor. Don't let Paul's advice frighten you into becoming a landlubber. This book is intended to keep you safe and healthy on the water . . . and even encourage you to range farther from the beach with more confidence. And Paul is an ideal captain for such a task.

I have already asked for several copies of *The Waterlover's*

Guide to Marine Medicine. I want one on my boat . . . and one in my tackle box . . . and a few copies for my children . . . just in case I have another grandchild flop down on a jellyfish and no one knows what to do.

Vin T. Sparano, Editor-in-Chief
Outdoor Life Magazine

PREFACE

I spent many hours as a boy watching my grandfather create intricate models of clipper ships, schooners, brigs, barks, and other sailing vessels. He served as mate or master on many of these ships and worked as a master rigger in Boston Harbor for many years after he retired from the sea, so the models were accurate in every detail, down to the last brace, jackstay, and buntline. I was always fascinated with the way he could take a few spools of thread and reconstruct the rigging from memory, and then explain to me how this intricate web of rope, blocks, and spars could be manipulated to drive the vessel to the far corners of the earth. As I watched my grandfather work, I would listen with rapt attention as he told me spellbinding stories of his days before the mast. Little wonder that I dreamed of one day becoming a sailor myself and commanding my own square-rigger as it sailed across the seas to distant and exotic lands.

It wasn't until I was a few years older, after my father started to tell me of his experiences as a merchant seaman before and during World War II, that I realized that life at sea wasn't all romance and adventure. I began to understand that a mariner's life was often hard and lonely. My interest in a career at sea faded and was replaced by a new-found fascination with medicine. I studied pre-med in college but retained enough interest in the sea to have spent the summer after my freshman year as a deckhand on an oil tanker. I loved the ship and being at sea, and I enjoyed being part of the crew. The men seemed to take a liking to me, and the bosun and cook nursed me back to health when I became seasick off Cape Hatteras. But, to a man, they encouraged me to stay in college, get my degree, and go on to medical school. I did, of course.

Part of the allure of medicine for me has been the intricate networks of nerves, blood vessels, muscles, tendons, and ligaments that comprise the human body. I marvel at the way that all these body components and the various organs work as beautifully coordinated systems to make the "vessel" think, feel, love, fight, work, play, create, and procreate. I believe that my fascination with complex but beautiful systems was kindled during those wonderful hours when I sat in my grandfather's kitchen overlooking Boston Harbor, watching him magically transform blocks of wood and spools of thread into miniature versions of the glorious sailing vessels he knew and loved so well as a younger man.

Boating enthusiasts are, as a group, nuts-and-bolts people who want to know how things work and enjoy using their analytical skills to solve problems. With that in mind, in this guide I have gone beyond the simple "signs, symptoms, treatment" formula and have explained *how* the various illnesses and injuries disrupt the normal anatomy and physiology. I trust the reader will find this approach more satisfying than a cookbook-style catalog of maladies and stock treatments.

The book is organized in a general-to-specific way. Chapter 1 deals with shock, cardiac arrest, and airway emergencies, and Chapters 2–6 address injuries to the various organ systems. Chapters 7–19 deal with specific marine medical problems. Treatment strategies discussed in the latter chapters presume a familiarity with the principles and techniques discussed in earlier chapters. Chapter 20 describes a ship's medical kit.

The best way to use this book is to read Chapter 1 first so that you'll have an idea what to do when confronted with an on-board life-and-death emergency. Then, I suggest that you follow the guidelines in Chapter 20 and put together a medical kit appropriate to your needs. You should read Chapters 8, 9, 10, 11, and 19 before your next cruise. The information contained in these sections pertains to *all* mariners, whatever their usual cruising grounds. You can read the remaining chapters whenever you have some slack time.

Keep the book in an easy-to-find place on board your boat, such as inside the medical kit or on the bookshelf at your navigation station.

The Waterlover's Guide to Marine Medicine covers most of the problems you're likely to encounter at sea, but at times you may need more detailed advice. You can get medical advice over the airways by calling the Coast Guard on VHF channel 16, and then continuing your communications on channel 22.

If you are beyond VHF range and have a single sideband (SSB) radio, make your call on MF 2182 kHz (a monitored frequency) or one of the HF frequencies and then switch to 2670 kHz. (The modulation is J3E for American vessels in United States waters and H3E for transmissions to ships and foreign-shore stations.)

DH MEDICO

DEADHEAD (DH) MEDICO is a free radio medical advice service available to mariners anywhere on the seven seas at any time of day or night. A doctor at the International Radio Medical Center (CIRM) in Rome will recommend treatment, consult specialists when indicated, guide you until the patient recovers, or arrange for evacuation or transfer to a vessel carrying a ship's doctor.

If you need assistance, try to make direct contact with the nearest call station. If you don't know its call signal, call NCG (any Coast Guard station). Use VHF Channel 16 or 2182 kHz SSB, or one of the HF frequencies set aside for distress and safety communications for DH MEDICO. When you are in American waters and need *urgent* medical advice, prefix your transmission with the "urgent" signal (XXX XXX XXX) and DH MEDICO.

If you experience language difficulties while using DH MED-

ICO, you can transcribe your messages into the Medical Signal Code of the International Code of Signals.

I have many physician colleagues who sail. For them, and for the many other boating enthusiasts with formal medical training, whether they be nurses, emergency medical technicians, or physician's assistants, I have described treatment recommendations for various disorders that involve fairly sophisticated medical procedures, such as starting intravenous lines, debriding wounds, and performing chest decompression to relieve tension pneumothorax. I realize that these are potentially dangerous interventions, but in a tight situation, on a boat at sea, hours or days from medical help, one's ability to perform such procedures may spell the difference between life and death.

I would strongly urge medical people who cruise offshore to take the American College of Surgeons' Advanced Trauma Life Support Course offered at many hospitals around the country. I would also recommend that you keep a copy of *Emergency Medicine: A Comprehensive Study Guide* on board. You can buy a copy by calling the American College of Emergency Physicians at (800) 798-1822.

Paul G. Gill, Jr., M.D.
Middlebury, Vermont
September 1992

SHOCK, AIRWAY EMERGENCIES, AND CPR

Shamrock *was running wing and wing down the Strait of Magellan before a strong northwesterly breeze when the williwaw struck. The Cape Horn snorter came roaring down out of the ice-capped mountains of Tierra del Fuego, whipped the indigo waters of the strait into a frothing frenzy, and blasted the 45-foot ketch with 80-knot winds. The first gust ripped the jib and mizzen to shreds, hurled the main boom across the deck like a giant scythe, and heaved the boat over onto her beam ends.* Shamrock *had barely recovered from the knockdown when a mountainous, 50-foot wave came barreling down the strait, tilted her stern spreader-high, and thrust her headlong down its steep front slope. She surfed deep into the trough of the wave, submarined her foredeck, and was sent flying stern-over-bow by the following crest.*

The helmsman clung to the steering wheel with a death grip during Shamrock's *terrifying ride down the front of the wave. When the yacht pitchpoled, the impact smashed him against the wheel, crushing his chest and bending the wheel like a pretzel. Two men were thrown over the side and dragged along under the hull by their tethers. Another was slammed belly-first against the sampson post.*

The rest of the crew were in the galley eating supper when the williwaw struck. They were thrown out of their seats and pummeled by a torrent of crashing lamps, jars, cans, blocks, shackles, frying pans, crockery, and instruments. They lay, stunned and battered, on the ceiling of the main cabin, listening with horror in the inky darkness as seawater poured in through the companionway hatch, air vents, and cockpit seats.

After a few seconds, the massive lead keel swung down and righted the ketch. The walking wounded fought their way topside through the debris, started the pumps, cleared the wreckage from the deck, and got the ketch under way. They ran downwind under bare poles for a few minutes, then entered a sheltered fjord, anchored, and turned their attention to their injured crewmates.

MASS CASUALTIES

OK, Skipper, what do you do now? You're holed up in a fjord in Tierra del Fuego in a violent storm, and you've got eight people on board a battered yacht, with an assortment of injuries.

If your vessel isn't named the SS *Hope,* you are not going to have the wherewithal to do more than stabilize the injured and arrange for them to be evacuated to a mainland hospital. If you are cruising in Penobscot Bay or in the waters off San Diego, help from the U.S. Coast Guard is only a radio call away. But if you are in the Strait of Magellan, the Doldrums, or midway between St. Helena and Tristan da Cunha in the South Atlantic when disaster strikes, you are going to be skipper *and* ship's doctor for several hours or days. You'll do fine if you maintain your composure, administer to the sick and injured in a humane and compassionate manner, and obey the Golden Rule of medicine: "First, do no harm."

Triage

The first thing you must do is *triage* (sort) the victims into three groups:

1. Those who will survive whether they are treated or not.

2. Those who have life-threatening injuries that require immediate attention.

3. Those who will die no matter what you do for them.

Then, focus your attention on the victims who fall into the second category.

SHOCK

The human body . . . indeed is like a ship; its bones being the stiff standing-rigging, and the sinews the small running ropes, that manage all the motions.

—Herman Melville, *Redburn*

When a warship receives a hit in its vitals, the captain sounds "General Quarters" and orders damage-control parties into action. They attempt to keep the vessel afloat and in the fight by sealing watertight compartments, maintaining buoyancy and stability, putting out fires, repairing or restoring damaged equipment, supplying emergency power, and administering first aid to the injured.

When you take a hit in *your* vitals, whether it be a large, bleeding wound, crushed chest, ruptured internal organs, extensive burns, or multiple fractures, your body also goes to "general quarters." Every organ system participates in an all-out effort to limit and repair the damage and keep the body "afloat." If you lose so much blood or plasma that you cannot maintain adequate blood flow to the vital organs, you go into *shock*.

Shock is the breakdown of vital functions that follows collapse of the circulation. Circulatory collapse can be secondary to extensive bleeding (*hemorrhagic shock*); severe fluid loss from extensive burns, crush injuries, or protracted vomiting and diarrhea (*hypovolemic shock*); heart failure (*cardiogenic shock*); severe allergic reactions (*anaphylactic shock*); overwhelming infection (*septic shock*); or fainting (*neurogenic shock*). Every cell in your body must receive a steady supply of oxygen and nutrients from the blood, and must be able to discharge carbon dioxide and other wastes into the blood. If circulatory collapse persists for more than an hour, cellular metabolism fails, and shock becomes irreversible and death inevitable.

Battle Stations

The *Shamrock* crewman who was slammed into the sampson post ruptured his spleen, bled internally, and went into shock. This is how his body responded: Pressure sensors in the large arteries in his chest and neck detected a drop in blood pressure and transmitted this information to the *vasomotor area* of the brain, the body's damage-control center. The vasomotor area acted swiftly to stabilize the circulation by stimulating the *sympathetic nervous system* (SNS), a special network of nerves supplying the heart and blood vessels. The SNS then:

1. Made the heart beat harder and faster.

2. Constricted large veins throughout the body, producing an "autotransfusion" of 5 pints of blood into the injured man's main circulation.

3. Constricted the arteries in the muscles, intestines, skin, and kidneys, diverting blood from these areas to the brain and heart.

At the same time, his kidneys started conserving salt and water, and fluid in the tissue spaces moved into the blood vessels. Both of these mechanisms helped to increase his circulating blood volume.

When the Royal Navy brought the German battleship *Bismarck* to bay in the North Atlantic in May 1940, the *Bismarck* continued to fight even after having been battered by more than four hundred direct hits with 16-inch and smaller shells and several torpedoes. Her tough armor, strong, watertight bulkheads, redundant communications, and superb damage-control systems kept her afloat long after any lesser ship would have gone to the bottom.

The human body's damage-control systems are also very efficient. So efficient, in fact, that a twenty-year-old can lose 2 to 4 pints of blood (25 to 30 percent of his blood volume) and show no outward sign of shock other than a rapid pulse and cool, moist skin. However, he is poised on the edge of disaster; if he loses even a few more cc's of blood, he may go into progressive and irreversible shock.

Recognizing Shock

Time, tide, and *shock* wait for no man. Shock must be recognized quickly and treated aggressively. If it is not reversed within one hour, the patient will die.

Here's what the shock victim looks like:

• *Mild Shock.* There is a blood loss of up to 2 pints. The body is compensating well, and blood pressure remains normal. The victim is alert but cold and thirsty; he may feel weak and lightheaded when he sits up. His pulse is rapid (110 to 120 beats a minute) and his skin is pale, cool, and damp.

• *Moderate shock.* The victim has lost 2 to 5 pints of blood; he is thirsty and short of breath, and unable to help himself. His speech is slurred, his skin is cold and clammy, his pulse is very rapid and thready, and his urine output meager (less than 30 mL per hour).

• *Severe shock.* The victim has lost half or more of his blood volume (5 pints plus) and the circulation to his heart and brain is poor. His eyes are dull and glazed, his pupils dilated, his breathing shallow and rapid. He becomes restless and agitated, and then lethargic and comatose.

Fighting Shock

When treating a trauma victim, proceed in an orderly fashion as follows.

1. First, tend to the ABCs.

a. Airway. If he is unconscious, use the jaw-thrust technique to open his airway: Put your fingers under each side of his jaw and lift it up and forward *without tilting his head back* (see Figure 1).

b. Breathing. Listen to his mouth and chest and observe his chest and abdomen. If you see chest and abdominal movement but don't hear breath sounds, check the airway again. If you still don't hear breath sounds, give two quick mouth-to-mouth breaths and go on to C.

c. Circulation. Put your index and middle fingers over the windpipe and slide them down alongside the neck muscle to feel for a pulse. If you don't feel one, start cardiopulmonary resuscitation, i.e., CPR (see below).

2. Then, examine the victim from head to toe for other serious injuries. Treat head, neck, eye, chest, or abdominal injuries as described in Chapters 3 and 4. Splint obvious fractures and dislocations (see Chapter 5). Controlling arterial bleeding can be like trying to douse a chute in a hurricane. Apply steady, firm pressure directly over the wound for a few minutes with a sterile bandage or any reasonably clean material. If the bleeding continues, pack the wound with sterile gauze and then cover it with a compression dressing. To control severe bleeding from a leg wound, drive your fist into the abdomen at the level of the navel to compress the aorta against the spinal column while an assistant applies a bulky compression dressing to the bandage.

3. After you have done everything you can to stabilize his injuries, place the victim on his back with his legs bent at the hips, knees straight, feet elevated 12 inches, and head down (the shock position). This position combats shock by promoting the return of venous blood to the heart. (Keep his head level if he

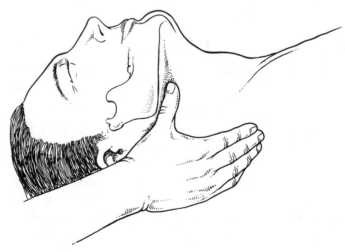

FIGURE 1
Opening the airway with the jaw-thrust technique.

has a head injury and place him in a semi-supine position if he has a chest injury.)

4. Cover him with blankets and offer him warm fluids by mouth if he is alert. If you are medically trained, start two large-bore (16 gauge) peripheral intravenous lines and infuse lactated Ringer's solution at a wide-open rate until the vital signs stabilize.

5. Carefully carry him down into the cabin if it is cold and wet topside. Check his vital signs, including his pulse and breathing rate and pattern, every few minutes. (Remember, agitation is a sign of deepening shock.)

6. Get on the radio and call for help.

TOURNIQUETS

Tourniquets are double-edged swords. They can be life-saving, but they can also irreparably damage muscles, nerves and blood vessels.

CAUTION! Don't apply a tourniquet unless you are prepared to write off the limb to save the victim.

You can make a tourniquet by folding a triangular bandage or a long strip of cloth into a band 2 inches wide. Here's how to apply it:

1. Place the tourniquet just above the wound; circle the limb with it twice; then tie the ends in an overhand knot.

2. Make a Spanish windlass by placing a 6-inch piece of wood over the knot and tying it in place with a square knot.

3. Rotate the windlass until the bleeding stops; then tie it in place with the free ends of the tourniquet.

4. On a tag, record the date and time the tourniquet was applied and pin it to the victim's clothing. Keep the tourniquet exposed and don't release it unless advised to do so by a physician or by emergency medical personnel.

CHOKING

Acute airway obstruction is the most serious of medical emergencies. If you are sitting in the galley eating dinner one evening and your mate suddenly turns blue and grabs his throat, it's not your cooking. He's having a "cafe coronary," which is simply a colorful way of saying that he is choking on a piece of food and will die of asphyxiation if you don't perform the Heimlich maneuver on him real quick.

If he is talking or coughing and spluttering, *leave him alone!* His airway is only *partially* blocked. Encourage him to cough out the food, but don't slap him on the back or perform the Heimlich maneuver.

If he turns blue and starts to make a high-pitched, screechy noise when he breathes, the obstruction is nearly complete. If he can't talk and clutches his throat with his hands (the universal distress signal), the obstruction is complete. In either case, it's time for you to perform the *Heimlich maneuver.* This is a series of abdominal thrusts that elevate the diaphragm and cause a sudden elevation of the pressure inside the chest cavity and an artificial cough that expels the foreign object. Here are the American Heart Association's recommendations for treating the choking victim.

1. *The victim is standing or sitting, and conscious.* Stand behind him and wrap your arms around his waist. Make a fist with one hand, and place the thumb side of the fist against his abdomen, just above the navel. Grab your fist with your other hand and press it into his abdomen with a quick, upward thrust (see Figure 2). Continue the thrusts until the airway is cleared or he loses consciousness. If he does lose consciousness, perform a finger sweep: Open his mouth by grasping the tongue and lower jaw and lifting up. Then, insert the index finger of your other hand alongside the cheek to the base of the tongue. Hook the finger behind the object and remove it from the mouth. (Be careful not to push the object deeper into the throat!) Then, give a series of mouth-to-mouth breaths. If you can't ventilate the lungs, perform six to ten abdom-

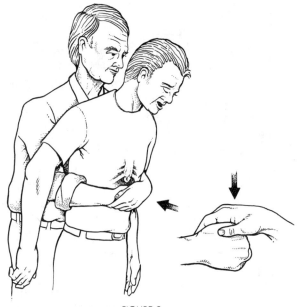

FIGURE 2
The Heimlich maneuver.

inal thrusts; repeat the finger sweep and the mouth-to-mouth ventilations. Repeat the sequence of Heimlich maneuver, finger sweep, and mouth-to-mouth breathing until the airway is cleared.

2. *The victim is lying on the ground unconscious.* Place him in a supine position, and kneel astride his thighs. Place the heel of one hand against his abdomen just above the navel, and put the other hand over the first. Press into the abdomen with a quick upward thrust. Repeat the Heimlich maneuver, finger sweep, ventilation sequence as necessary. (You can use this technique on the conscious choking victim if your arms are too short to reach around his waist.)

3. *The victim is very obese or pregnant, and conscious.* Stand behind the victim, and wrap your arms around his or her chest. Place the thumb side of your fist on the middle of the breastbone, grab your fist with the other hand, and perform a series of backward thrusts until the airway is cleared or the victim loses consciousness.

4. *The victim is very obese or pregnant, and unconscious.* Place the victim on his or her back, kneel alongside him or her, and place the heel of your hand on the lower half of the breastbone. Place the other hand over the first, and perform a series of thrusts. As above, repeat Heimlich maneuvers, finger sweeps, and ventilations until the airway is cleared.

5. *The choking victim is an infant.* If you are sure that the child is choking on an object, and not suffering from a severe upper respiratory infection, position the child head down so that he is straddling your forearm, and deliver four brisk blows between the shoulder blades with the heel of your hand. Then turn the infant face-up, position it on your thigh with its head down, and perform four chest thrusts, as described above.

6. *You are alone and choking.* Perform the Heimlich maneuver on yourself. Make a fist with one hand, and place the thumb side on the abdomen just above the navel. Grab the fist with the other hand, and press inward and upward in a quick, sharp, thrusting motion. If this doesn't work, press your abdomen across any firm surface, such as the steering wheel, air vent, or outboard motor.

WARNING! When doing abdominal or chest thrusts, be careful not to place your fist too near the xiphoid (the bony projection at the bottom of the breastbone) or on the lower ribs. Fractures of the xiphoid or ribs can lacerate the liver, spleen, or lungs. And position the victim with his head lower than his trunk so that he won't regurgitate and aspirate his stomach contents.

CARDIOPULMONARY RESUSCITATION (CPR)

Would you know what to do if your mate collapsed on deck with an apparent heart attack? You certainly wouldn't want to pull on his tongue, stretch his rectum, or bury him up to his chest and splash water on his face. Fortunately, those resuscitation methods are no longer recommended. But CPR is, and you should become proficient in it by taking a Basic Life Support (BLS) course. A review of the techniques follows on page 27.

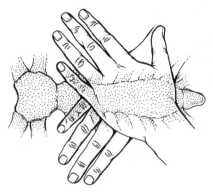

FIGURE 3
Proper hand position for chest compression.

1. *Airway.* Establish that the victim is unresponsive, place him on his back on a firm, flat surface, and open his airway using the jaw-thrust technique.

2. *Breathing.* Kneel alongside the victim, and check to see if he is breathing by watching for movement of his chest and abdomen and listening for breath sounds with your ear against his mouth and nose. If he is not breathing, perform mouth-to-mouth breathing by pinching his nostrils, taking a deep breath, sealing your lips around his mouth, and giving him two full breaths.

3. *Circulation.* Check his neck for pulses and, if absent, do chest compressions as follows.

a. Place the heel of one hand on the lower half of the breast bone, and place your other hand over the first (see Figure 3).

b. Keeping your shoulders over his chest and your elbows locked, compress the chest at a rate of 60 per minute, stopping every 15 compressions to open the airway and give two breaths (see Figure 4). The breastbone should be depressed 1.5 to 2 inches with each compression.

CAUTION! Excessively forceful or misplaced compressions can cause fractures and injuries to internal organs. Don't let the heel of your hand slide down over xiphoid, and keep your fingers away from the chest.

Continue CPR until:

1. Breathing and pulses return.

2. The rescuers are exhausted.

3. The rescuers are in danger.

4. The victim fails to respond to prolonged resuscitation (hypothermia victims may respond after lengthy CPR).

5. You are relieved by medical professionals.

CPR shouldn't be attempted in the following situations.

1. A lethal injury, when imminent death is obvious.

2. A dangerous setting where rescuers would be jeopardizing their own lives.

3. Chest compressions are impossible, e.g., the chest is frozen or crushed.

4. When any breathing or movement is evident.

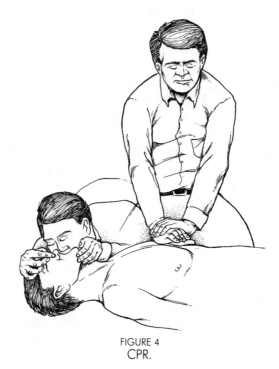

FIGURE 4
CPR.

·
·
·
·
·

2

SOFT-TISSUE INJURIES AND BURNS

"Jerry" the Greek, whose leg had been smashed to pulp when caught in the washport . . . was lashed into his own bunk in the forecastle, and was suffering immeasurable torments, as gangrene had set in.

"Dere ist only von t'ing to save him der life," growled Gronberg. "Cut him der leg off, or he die pretty quick!"

"What's that you say?" said Captain Barker, a man who never shirked a tough decision; and, after considering a moment: "By heavens, I think you're right! I'll do it!"

—W. H. S. Jones, The Cape Horn Breed

Skin is stretchable, waterproof, and tattooable, but it's not very tough. I'm painfully reminded of how fragile my skin is every time I dive on a coral reef or bump my shoulder against the barnacle-encrusted piling next to my slip. But cuts, abrasions, splinters, and embedded fishhooks are a way of life for mariners. If you don't own a Teflon bodysuit, you'd better learn how to treat these injuries at sea.

OPEN WOUNDS

Open wounds are breaks in the skin, the body's first line of defense against bacteria, viruses, and other germs. There are several types of open wounds, and they range in seriousness from abrasions to amputations.

Assessment and Treatment

Pointers on how to treat open wounds follow on page 30.

Control the Bleeding

Even the most severe bleeding will stop if you apply firm pressure to the wound. After a few minutes, the ends of the cut vessels constrict, and a clot forms and plugs the hole in the vessel. Tourniquets are rarely necessary and are fraught with hazard (see Chapter 1).

Inspect the Wound

Once you get the bleeding under control, wash your hands and inspect the wound. Determine how deep it is, and check for damage to bones, tendons, ligaments, and blood vessels. If the wound is on the arm or leg, check the pulses at the wrist or ankle (see "A Systematic Approach to Skeletal Injuries" in Chapter 5), and determine whether the victim has sensation below the wound and full movement of his hands, fingers, feet, and toes.

Clean the Wound

First, use a pair of tissue forceps or tweezers to pick out any foreign matter that may be present. Next, use a bulb syringe to thoroughly irrigate the wound with water or irrigating solution (add an ounce of 10% povidone-iodine solution to 2 or 3 quarts of water). Then, gently wipe dirt out of the wound with a sterile gauze pad.

Decide Whether to Close the Wound or Leave It Open

It's not necessary to close every wound. In fact, many wounds are best left open, especially if there is a high risk of infection, such as with fish bites and stings. No matter how meticulous you are in cleansing the wound, it's impossible to remove every contaminant when your operating theater is tossing and pitching and the operating table is your galley table. Bacteria thrive on the blood and necrotic debris that accumulate in the depths of cuts, so closing a deep, dirty gash is a recipe for infection. It's better to leave such wounds open so that pus can drain freely. But every injury has to be treated on its merits; the decision to close or not to close depends on its location and its depth, how badly it is contaminated, and whether there are associated bone, joint, tendon, or nerve injuries.

Abrasions

An abrasion is what you get when you scrape the skin over a bony prominence, such as your knee or elbow. The superficial layer of skin is sheared off, and dirt is often ground into the wound.

Treatment

Cleanse the abrasion with an antiseptic solution. Then cover it with a transparent dressing (Bioclusive or Tegaderm). Cover large abrasions with a multilayered bandage, and change the dressing daily until a firm scab forms.

Lacerations

A laceration is a wound made by tearing. Lacerations caused by knives or other sharp objects typically produce linear wounds with neat edges. Blunt trauma, such as results from striking your knee against the chart table in the dark or dropping an anchor on your foot, causes jagged, stellate lacerations.

Facial Lacerations

Facial lacerations can almost always be closed with tape skin closures. The rich blood supply of the face practically guarantees against infection, providing the wound is thoroughly cleansed. First, apply tincture of benzoin to the skin on either side of the wound to make the tapes adhere better, and spread antibiotic ointment on the wound. Then bring the wound edges together by applying a tape first to one side of the wound, and then the other. Make sure that there are no gaps in the wound and that the edges are even.

You can also use Super Glue (a cyanoacrylate) to close small, tension-free facial lacerations. Hold the wound edges together and squeeze enough glue onto the wound to cover the wound edges with a thin film, but don't let the glue penetrate into the wound. Then, maintain pressure on the wound until the glue dries (30 to 40 seconds). The glue is waterproof, so a dressing is unnecessary.

Scalp Lacerations

Bleeding from scalp wounds can be brisk and difficult to control. You can close the wound quickly and easily by tying clumps of hair across it until the bleeding stops. (Hair doesn't hold knots well, so use surgeon's knots—square knots with an extra throw.) Then apply a turban bandage using a roll of 4-inch roll gauze.

Trunk and Limb Lacerations

Trunk and limb lacerations should be cleansed, closed with surgical staples when appropriate, coated with antibiotic ointment, and covered with a multilayer sterile dressing. The first layer should be a nonabsorbent sterile dressing, such as Vaseline gauze (Adaptic). The next layer should consist of sterile gauze pads, followed by an ABD or Surgipad if the laceration is large. The dressings can then be taped down or wrapped with roll gauze.

Any small laceration on the trunk and limbs can be closed with Super Glue (see page 31). The glue may need to be reapplied periodically if the laceration is on a dynamic area, such as the elbow or back of the hand.

Avulsions

An avulsion is what you get when you whack off a piece of skin (usually a fingertip) with a knife or some other sharp object. In a partial-thickness avulsion, only the top layers of the skin are lost; a full-thickness avulsion involves loss of all of the skin and some of the underlying fatty layer.

You can't close avulsions, but you should still treat them as though they were lacerations. Skin will grow in from the sides and heal even the deepest of avulsions, providing bone isn't exposed. If it is, or if the avulsion is larger than a half-dollar, the wound will require skin grafting.

Avulsed skin that remains attached on one side is called a *flap*. Clean and dress a flap the way you would any other avulsion, but keep an eye on it. If it becomes infected, lift it off and start twice daily wet-to-dry dressings (see page 36).

Amputations

On large vessels, parting lines can whip through a man's legs like a hot knife through butter. Fingers and toes caught in a bight in an anchor rode or a halyard can be lopped off. But amputated fingers can often be saved if they are surgically reattached within 6 hours or so of injury.

Treatment
First, cleanse the stump and apply a bulky dressing. Then, wash the severed finger, wrap it in sterile gauze, put it in a container inside an ice chest, and head for the nearest hospital. (*CAU-TION!* Don't put the part directly on ice—the surgeon won't be able to reattach it if it is frostbitten.) If you are offshore, contact the Coast Guard and request helicopter transport to a medical facility with replantation capabilities. If you are more than 10 or 12 hours from land, and helicopter transport isn't available, treat the stump like any other open wound. It will have to be surgically revised when you make port.

Bleeding from an amputated limb can lead to shock and death if not quickly controlled. If you can't control the bleeding with firm compression on the stump, you'll have to apply a tourniquet (see Chapter 1).

PUNCTURE WOUNDS

Puncture wounds, no matter how minute, should never be ignored. It's never easy to estimate the depth of a puncture wound, but you should assume that the nail, splinter, or fish spine that caused it has driven bacteria and dirt deep into the tissues. It may even have punctured a blood vessel, nerve, tendon, or joint.

Treatment

Cleanse the wound thoroughly with antiseptic solution, and then cover it with antibiotic ointment and a bandage strip. If you haven't had a tetanus booster in 10 years, make sure you get one within 72 hours. (Puncture wounds produced by the spines of venomous fish require additional treatment as described in Chapter 17.)

How to Remove a Fishhook

Here are two ways to remove a fishhook.

The String Technique

1. Loop a 12-inch length of string around the curve of the hook, and wrap the ends around your index finger (see Figure 5).

2. Push down on the eye and shank of the hook with your free hand to disengage the barb.

3. Align the string with the shank's long axis. Then gently tug on the free ends of the string until the hook comes out through the entrance wound.

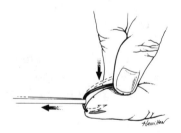

FIGURE 5
Fishhook removal using the string technique.

The Push-and-Snip Technique

1. If the barb is protruding through the skin, snip it off and back the hook out (see Figure 6).

2. If the barb *isn't* protruding, wash the skin around the wound with antiseptic solution, and then numb it with an ice cube. Grasp the shank of the hook with a pair of needle-nose pliers and push the point of the hook through the skin.

3. Snip off or flatten the barb, then back the hook out.

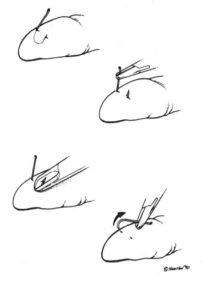

FIGURE 6
Fishhook removal using the push-and-snip technique.

After you remove the hook, treat the wound as you would any puncture wound.

Splinters

Removing embedded splinters can be tougher than freeing a fouled anchor.

Treatment
Focus a bright light on the wound, and make yourself comfortable. First, press gently on the skin around the entrance wound to get a feel for the orientation of the splinter. Then, put your finger against the deep end of the splinter and push it toward the en-

trance wound. Grasp the exposed portion of the splinter with your tweezers and pull it out. Then clean and dress the wound.

WET-TO-DRY DRESSINGS

A simple, but effective, way to treat dirty wounds is with wet-to-dry dressings. Cover the wound with wet, sterile, gauze pads, and change them twice a day after they dry out. Wet-to-dries control infection by removing pus and necrotic debris.

CONTUSIONS

Contusions are those bruises you get when you fall through an open hatch, or fall out of a bosun's chair and slam your elbow and hip against the cockpit coaming. They are crush injuries to the skin and underlying fat and muscle that become swollen and painful, and turn black and blue. Some deep contusions of the thigh or buttocks can be complicated by *hematomas,* collections of blood within the muscle. Blunt trauma to the tip of a finger can cause a hematoma under the nail *(subungual hematoma).*

Treatment
Treating contusions is as easy as RICE. That is Rest, Ice, Compression, and Elevation. Apply an ACE bandage to the contused limb, keep it elevated for 24 to 72 hours, apply ice for 15 minutes every 2 hours, and rest it as much as possible. Painful subungual hematomas can be drained if you are reasonably certain that the underlying bone isn't fractured. Here's the technique:

   1. Wash your hands with soap and water.
   2. Pull one end of a paper clip out to a 90-degree angle.
   3. Heat the tip of the clip over a flame until it is red hot. Then press it into the middle of and through the discolored area of the nail.

4. Withdraw the clip when blood drains from the nail.

5. When the nail stops draining, apply a bandage strip.

STRAINS

What happens when an irresistible force meets an immovable object? When the irresistible force is you and the immovable object is something heavy, such as an outboard motor, the result is frequently a muscle strain. A muscle strain, or pulled muscle, is an injury to the musculo-tendinous unit caused by sudden over-stretching of the muscle or a sudden increase in the tension within the unit. The muscle itself may tear, there may be a tear at the tendon-muscle junction, or the tendon may rupture or tear away from its bony origin or insertion.

Muscle strains fall into one of three categories, according to their severity.

A *grade I strain* is simply a tightening up of a muscle while you're straining to lift or push a heavy object. There are microscopic tears in the muscle fibers, but there is no defect in the muscle that you can see or feel.

If you feel a pop or snap while attempting to lift that outboard motor, you may have sustained a *grade II strain*. In this injury, up to 50 percent of the muscle fibers are torn, and there's an obvious defect in the muscle. You can still move the injured part, but there's a fair bit of pain and spasm.

Grade III strains are complete ruptures of the musculo-tendinous unit. These disabling injuries are heralded by a loud pop or snap and a surge of pain as the muscle or tendon ruptures or rips out of its bony insertion. In younger people, the tendon usually pulls away from the muscle, although it may tear out of its bony insertion, taking a fragment of bone with it. In older people, the tendon has lost some of its tensile strength and is the weakest link in the musculo-tendinous chain. You know you have a grade III muscle strain when you see or feel a large defect in the muscle and can't contract it normally, or when it's all bunched up, as in a ruptured hamstring or biceps tendon.

Treatment

Lots of RICE (see page 36) early in the course of the injury will prevent bleeding, swelling, and muscle spasm, and will minimize disability. The first thing you should do is splint the injured part in the position of maximum comfort. Then, put a soft pad over the injured muscle and wrap it in place with an Ace bandage. Keep the part elevated as much as possible over the next 24 to 72 hours, and apply ice for 15 minutes every 2 hours. A sling is a good idea for a strain of the shoulder or biceps. After two or three days of RICE, you can start soaking the injured part in a warm water bath. Gentle range-of-motion exercises will help prevent shortening and weakening of the healing muscles. You can expect grade I and most grade II strains to heal in a few days, but allow several weeks for recovery from more severe injuries. A grade III injury should be treated by a physician as soon as possible.

SPRAINS

Sprains are stretching, tearing injuries to *ligaments*, the thick, tough bands that stabilize the joints. When you slip on a wet deck and twist your knee or turn your ankle, the ligaments that support those joints will tear either partially (mild or moderate sprain, grade I or II) or completely (grade III). The joint will become swollen, painful, and black and blue. You'll barely be able to walk on a severe sprain, and the joint will feel as though it were going to give out.

Treatment

RICE (see page 36) is the formula, plus splinting when appropriate. Apply an elastic bandage or a splint to a sprained knee or ankle, and rest a sprained shoulder or elbow in a sling. Splint sprained wrists or hands in a "cock-up" splint by putting a balled-up pair of socks in the palm and splinting the wrist and hand to a 10-inch-long wooden or plastic slat. Sprained fingers should be buddy-taped to the adjoining finger. Remove the splint or elastic bandage in 24 to 48 hours and start warm soaks and gentle range-of-motion exercises. Be patient—sprains take several weeks to heal.

BURNS

You can sustain any type of burn (thermal, chemical, electrical, or friction) on shipboard, and you can treat most burns with the materials in your medical chest.

Evaluating Burns

Before treating a burn, estimate its depth, extent and severity.

Depth

First-degree Burns involve the *epidermis* (outer layer of the skin) only. The burned area is painful, red, and slightly swollen.

Second-degree Burns involve the epidermis and outer portion of the dermis (deep layer of the skin). The burned skin is red or white, and there may be many large blisters. These are exquisitely painful injuries.

Third-degree Burns destroy the epidermis and dermis and may extend to the fat, muscle, and bone. The skin is charred, or waxy and white; blood vessels can be seen through translucent areas. These burns are painless because the nerve endings are destroyed.

(*Note:* First- and second-degree burns are *partial-thickness* burns; third-degree burns are *full-thickness* burns.)

Extent

Use the "rule of nines" to estimate the extent of a burn (see Figure 7). The head and neck together represent 9 percent of the body surface area (BSA), the chest and back each 18 percent, each arm 9 percent, each leg 18 percent, and the genital area 1 percent. In children, the head represents up to 18 percent of BSA.

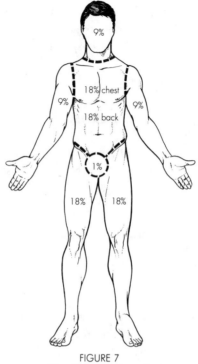

FIGURE 7
The "rule of nines."

Severity

Minor burns involve less than 15 percent BSA. *Moderate burns* involve 15 to 25 percent BSA. *Major burns* are burns involving more than 25 percent BSA or serious burns of hands, feet, or genitals; burns with associated injury (e.g., fractures or head injury); or burns in patients with severe preexisting medical problems (e.g., heart disease or diabetes).

Treatment

Minor and Moderate Burns

Cover small burns with cool or iced water. (*CAUTION!* Never apply ice directly to the burn. That only adds frostbite to a thermal injury.) Then, wash the burns with mild soap and water. Use a cotton ball to gently remove dirt and debris, and scissors and forceps to remove loose tissue and blisters (they contain chemicals which inhibit blood flow to the skin). Then apply a $1/16$-inch layer of silver sulfadiazine cream (antibiotic ointment on facial burns), and cover the burn with an occlusive gauze dressing or Spenco 2nd Skin. Bandage fingers and toes individually, and leave burns of the face, neck, and genitals uncovered. Remove the dressing once or twice daily, wash the burn with mild soap, and reapply the burn ointment and dressing. Partial-thickness burns heal within 7 to 10 days if they don't become infected. A tetanus booster is advised if more than five years have elapsed since the previous one.

Major Burns

Avoid panic and carry out the following procedures in sequence.

1. Quickly remove the victim from the fire and strip off any burning or smoldering clothing.

2. Tend to the ABCs (see Chapter 1) and stabilize life- or limb-threatening injuries as well as you can.

3. Check for other injuries.

4. Replace fluid losses. The massive loss of plasma from extensive burns can rapidly lead to shock. If you can, start an intravenous (IV) line and administer Ringer's lactate according to this formula:

2–4 cc/kg body weight/% BSA burn

Give one-half the amount in the first 8 hours, and one-half in the next 16 hours. If you can't start an IV, and the victim is conscious, have him drink half a glass of fluid every 15 minutes (give a child a quarter glass every 15 minutes).

5. Radio for help.

6. Give analgesics (by IV, preferably).

7. Wash the burns as described above. If dressings are in short supply, cover extensive burns with clean sheets.

8. Keep the victim supine (prone if burns are on the back) and warm while awaiting evacuation.

Electrical Burns

Electrical burns are notoriously difficult to evaluate because most of the damage is internal. There is an entrance wound and an exit wound, and there are varying degrees of thermal injury to the tissues traversed by the current, in direct proportion to their electrical resistance. Bones, muscles, blood vessels, and nerves usually are most seriously injured.

Treatment
First, remove the victim from the electrical source. Administer CPR if necessary. If not, treat the visible burns as outlined above, and give the victim plenty of fluids while awaiting evacuation to a hospital.

Chemical Burns

Acids, alkalis, and other chemicals can cause deceptively deep burns.

Treatment
Wash the exposed skin with copious amounts of water. Alkalis can produce deep, destructive ocular burns, so irrigate the eyes *extensively* if they are exposed to any chemical that you think might be alkaline, and report to the nearest hospital ASAP.

Friction Burns

If a gust of wind comes along and fills a doused spinnaker while you are holding the halyard, you might get a rope burn. This can range from a mild abrasion to a deep burn. Treat friction burns the same as other thermal burns. *Avoid* friction burns by keeping a couple of turns on the halyard winch when dropping the spinnaker and maintaining strain on a cleat or bitt when paying out the anchor rode.

·
·
·
·
·

3
HEAD, NECK, FACIAL, AND EYE INJURIES

*Groping blindly for the peak downhaul, I received a sharp
blow in the face, then my neck was encircled in a vice-like
grip and I soared aloft, caught in a bight of the downhaul
whipped about by the flailing gaff. I knew no more until I hit
the deck with a jarring shock. . . .*

—Captain Richard England, *Schoonerman*

Getting hoisted aloft by a downhaul or halyard is only one of the
many ways in which you can break your neck, crack your skull, or
break your jaw on a sailboat. You could just as easily be thrown
down the companionway by a wave breaking over the stern, or be
smashed in the head by a jibing boom.

HEAD INJURIES

What do you do when your shipmate is knocked senseless by a
comber that breaks over the side and slams him into the scuppers?
Drag him down into the cabin? Throw a bucket of cold water in
his face? You'd better not. If he has a serious head injury, cold
water isn't going to revive him. And if he has a broken neck,
you could cause permanent paralysis by moving him without first
splinting his cervical spine.

Approach the head-injury victim the way you would approach
any trauma victim: First tend to the ABCs (Airway, Breathing,
and Circulation), and then do a quick head-to-toe exam.
CAUTION! Keep the neck rigidly immobilized until you are certain it isn't injured!

Then evaluate the head injury more thoroughly by checking
the following on page 44.

1. *Eye opening.* Does he open his eyes spontaneously, on command, or only in response to pain?
2. *Verbal response.* Can you understand his speech, or is it gibberish? Does he make sense, or is he confused and disoriented?
3. *Motor response.* Does he obey simply commands? If not, does he withdraw from a painful stimulus?
4. *Pupillary responses.* Are his pupils round and symmetrical? Do they constrict when you shine a light into his eyes?

Based on these responses, assign your crewmate's head injury to one of these categories.

Concussion

If he wakes up after a short while and acts a little groggy, but can talk and walk normally, he has probably had a simple *concussion,* which is a transient disruption of brain function. He may not remember how he got hurt, and he may have a headache and difficulty concentrating for a few days, but he'll be OK.

Intracranial Bleeding

If he remains unconscious, or wakes up for a short period and then lapses into a coma, he probably has *intracranial bleeding;* i.e., bleeding between the brain and the skull (*epidural* or *subdural hematoma*—see Figure 8) or bleeding within the substance of the brain (*intracerebral bleeding*). Intracranial bleeding is a life-threatening emergency. Since the brain is encased in the skull, which is rigid and can't expand, intracranial bleeding causes the pressure within the head to increase. When the pressure exceeds a critical level, blood flow to the brain stops, and the brain cells die. There's nothing you can do to reverse the situation on shipboard, so if you believe that your shipmate has intracranial bleeding, get on the radio immediately and request helicopter evacuation to a hospital.

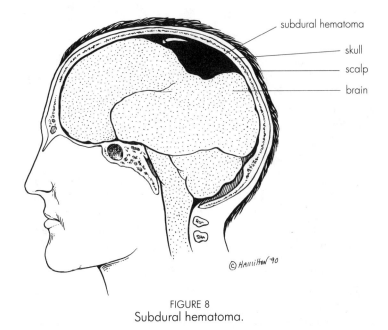

subdural hematoma

skull

scalp

brain

© Hamilton '90

FIGURE 8
Subdural hematoma.

SKULL FRACTURE

A bruise behind the ear, "raccoon eyes," bleeding from the ears, and drainage of clear fluid from the nose or ears are all signs of a *basilar skull fracture* (fracture of the base of the skull). If your shipmate has a scalp laceration, wash your hands thoroughly or slip on a pair of sterile gloves and carefully explore the wound. Is there a skull defect? Is the brain exposed? If there is no obvious open brain injury, run your finger over the surface of the skull. If you feel a depression, your mate has a *depressed skull fracture*. A skull fracture in its own right is not life-threatening, but it may be complicated by underlying brain injury or intracranial bleeding and is grounds for immediate evacuation to a hospital. Don't make any attempt to clean an open skull fracture, and *never* pull a penetrating object out of the skull. Just apply a sterile dressing and a turban bandage and keep the victim warm while awaiting evacuation.

NECK INJURIES

Neck injuries follow head trauma as surely as the anchor chain follows the anchor. If your shipmate tumbles head-first down an open hatch, or falls out of the bosun's chair and lands in a heap on the deck, you must assume that he has a neck injury. If he has a spinal injury and you attempt to move him, bone fragments could penetrate the spinal cord and cause paralysis or death.

If you are sailing into the teeth of a Force 7 gale and monstrous seas are crashing over the bows and sweeping the deck, you are naturally going to be anxious to move the victim into the cabin. But before you grab him by the ankles and start dragging him aft, do the following.

1. If he is conscious, ask him if his neck or back hurts. If he says no and he can move his head comfortably in all directions, he probably doesn't have a significant neck injury.

2. Next, run your fingers down his spinal column from the base of his skull to his tailbone and feel for irregularities or tenderness.

3. If head movement is painful or his spine is tender, have an assistant support his head while you wrap a rolled-up bath towel snugly around his neck and secure it with safety pins or adhesive tape. Then, while keeping his neck in neutral position (neither flexed nor extended), *gently* move him onto a long board or a pair of lashed oars and secure him to the board or lashed oars with straps or tape. Stuff two duffle bags with clothing or linen, apply one to each side of his head, and secure them in place with one or two long strips of tape running from one side of the board, across his forehead, and under the other side of the board (see Figure 9). If you don't have small duffle bags, use a couple of small fenders or hardcover books. (If you believe he has a back injury, keep him in a supine position.) Now you can safely move him to the cabin.

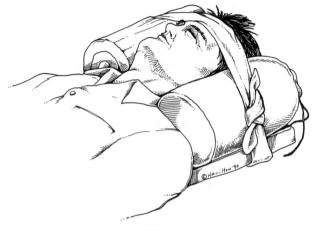

FIGURE 9
Immobilizing the neck.

Detecting Spinal Cord Injuries

After you have immobilized the victim's spine and gotten him out of the weather, look for these signs of *spinal cord injury.*

1. Neck or back pain radiating down the arms or legs.

2. Numbness or tingling in the hands or feet.

3. Complete or partial loss of feeling in the arms or legs (he may be able to feel pressure or hot and cold, but not pain).

4. Weakness or paralysis of the arms or legs.

5. A sustained penile erection.

6. Inability to urinate.

Anyone with a suspected spinal cord injury needs to be promptly evacuated to a hospital. Have someone get on the radio and make arrangements while you tend to any other injuries he may have. Offer him aspirin or acetaminophen if he is alert, and keep him warm. Pressure sores can develop in a few hours in a spinal cord patient, so put some padding under his elbows, buttocks, and heels. If he vomits, carefully log-roll him onto his side so that he doesn't aspirate the vomitus.

FACIAL INJURIES

Here is a catalogue of the facial injuries you might sustain on shipboard.

Blowout Fracture

If a shipmate gets hit in the eye by a small block or an oar handle moving at high speed, the sudden increase in pressure can blow out the thin floor of his eye socket (see Figure 10). Following a blowout fracture, the eyeball may have a sunken-in appearance; but it rarely ruptures, and vision is generally preserved. He'll have a shiner, swollen eyelids, swelling and tenderness over the upper cheek, and possibly double or blurred vision and numbness of the cheek and upper lip.

Treatment
Blowout fractures require the tender mercies of a plastic surgeon ASAP. While returning to port, apply a large ice pack to the

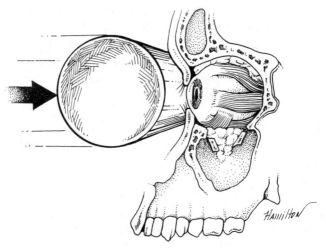

FIGURE 10
Blow-out fracture of the orbit.

injured area, and give analgesics as needed. If the eye appears to be injured, cover it with a metal shield.

Fractured Jaw

The mandible (jawbone) is one of the strongest bones in the body, but it's no match for a jibing boom or a swinging spinnaker pole. Other than pain, the first thing the victim will notice after breaking his jaw is that his bite is "off." He'll feel *crepitus* (a "crunchy" sensation) when he opens or closes his mouth, and his jaw may look asymmetric. There may also be a bruise in the floor of the mouth near the fracture site or sites and numbness of the lower lip and chin.

Treatment
Remove any loose teeth and have the victim rinse his mouth with water. Then splint the fracture by wrapping a muslin cravat (bandage) around his head and under the jaw. If he is bleeding from the mouth, the fracture is probably open (i.e., there is a deep wound over the fracture site and the fracture fragments are exposed.) Administer penicillin V potassium (penicillin VK), 250 mg every 6 hours. Fractured mandibles require operative fixation, so get him to a hospital quickly.

Dislocated Jaw

You don't have to be smashed in the face to dislocate your jaw. A hard tap on the chin can do it, but so can yawning, or just opening your mouth wide. The victim will get intense pain and swelling over one or both of the *TMJs* (temporomandibular joints), where the mandible forms a ball-and-socket joint with the temporal bone just in front of the ear. He'll have trouble talking and swallowing, and his jaw will be locked open and protrude outward, or deviate to one side.

Treatment

Here's how to reduce a dislocated jaw:

1. Wrap your thumbs in 4″ x 4″ gauze.

2. Place them on the back, lower molar teeth; then curl your fingers under the jaw.

3. Press downward on the molars while the mouth is opened wide.

4. Push the chin backward until the condyles snap back into the joint sockets.

Keep your patient on a soft diet for a few days, give him a mild analgesic as needed, and warn him not to open his jaw wide or yawn for at least two weeks.

Nasal injuries

> . . . the two brutes picked up the senseless man like a sack of rubbish and hove him clear up the companion stairs, through the narrow doorway, and out on deck. The blood from his nose gushed in a scarlet stream over the feet of the helmsman. . . .

—Jack London, The Sea Wolf

If your nose is fractured, and not just bruised, you'll detect crepitus and hypermobility when you squeeze the bridge, and you may have a nosebleed and deformity as well. You may be able to mold the fracture fragments into good alignment with your fingers, but if your nose appears misshapen, you'll have to consult an otolaryngologist (ear, nose, and throat specialist), preferably within a week of the injury. Ice will help control swelling, and analgesics may be required.

Any hard blow to the nose can cause a *septal hematoma*. This is a grapelike nodule that forms on the septum, the cartilage plate in the center of your nose. Untreated, it can lead to a septal abscess or necrosis and deformity of the septum.

Treatment

A septal hematoma should normally be treated by an otolaryngologist, but if you are westing through the Denmark Strait, you're going to have to do it yourself. First, swab the septum with antiseptic solution. Then, use a No. 11 scalpel to make a small, vertical incision in the hematoma so that it can drain. Finally, coat the nasal membrane with antibiotic ointment, and pack the nose with strips of gauze to keep firm pressure on the hematoma. Administer amoxicillin, 250 mg every 8 hours, and remove the packing in three days.

You can get most *nosebleeds* to stop by having the victim lean forward and squeeze the soft part of his nose for 5 or 10 minutes. If that doesn't do it, have him clear his nose. Then use a penlight to try to identify the bleeding site. Usually, it will be in Kiesselbach's area, an area in the front part of the septum where there is a rich supply of blood vessels (see Figure 11). Once you have found the bleeding site, cauterize it with a silver nitrate stick. If the bleeding persists, pack the nose and administer antibiotics, as described above. If blood is draining down the back of the throat, and you can't find a bleeding site, the victim may have a *posterior*

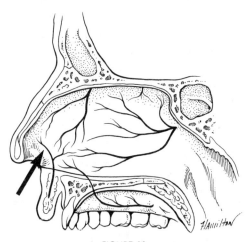

FIGURE 11
Kiesselbach's area.

nosebleed. The only thing you can do in that case is to get him to medical help ASAP.

EYE INJURIES

Some of the eye injuries you may have to treat on shipboard include the following.

Corneal Injuries

The cornea is the most sensitive area of the body, so it's little wonder that a tiny grain of sand in your eye can feel like a harpoon. Fortunately, corneal pain triggers a flood of tears that usually washes out sand and other foreign bodies. However, a foreign object may get caught under the upper lid and scrape the cornea each time you open and close your eyelid, causing a painful *corneal abrasion*.

Treatment
If sand or grit gets into your shipmate's eye, sit him down under a good light, instill one drop of Tetracaine solution to anesthetize the cornea, and then examine the eye. Observe the shape and symmetry of the pupils, and check his visual acuity by asking him to read newsprint (if he wears glasses, test his acuity with his glasses on). Examine the cornea and *sclera* (the white of the eye) with a magnifying glass, looking for scratched areas (abrasions) or embedded foreign bodies. Then use a Q-tip cotton swab or a matchstick to evert the upper lid, and inspect the recess under the everted lid.

If you see a foreign object, try to flush it out with a gentle stream of clean water. If that fails, try pulling the lid down over the lashes of the lower lid. As a final resort, try to gently lift the object off the cornea with a moistened Q-tip (see Figure 12).

Pain that persists after removal of a speck of sand is usually caused by a corneal abrasion. Instill one drop each of sulfacetamide 10% ophthalmic suspension and homatropine 2% solution

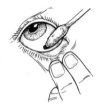

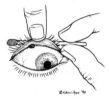

FIGURE 12
Removing a foreign body from the eye.

into the injured eye, and then apply a tight, double eye patch. (Fold one patch in half and place it over the closed eye. Then place the other patch over the folded patch and secure it with strips of adhesive tape.) Have the victim wear the patch for 12 to 24 hours. If his symptoms persist beyond 24 hours, and he remains convinced that there is an object in his eye, he's probably right. It just may be too small for you to see, or it may be hiding under the corner of the eyelid. Take another look; if you still can't see anything, he needs to see an ophthalmologist as soon as possible.

Blunt and Penetrating Injuries to the Eye

If you get poked in the eye with the end of a jibsheet, you may sustain only a *subconjunctival hemorrhage*. Small blood vessels in the sclera rupture and blood accumulates just beneath the *conjunctiva*, the translucent membrane that covers the eyeball. The eye looks terrible, but no treatment is necessary. The blood will disappear in about 14 days.

A crewmate who is struck in the eye by a cleat that has ripped out of the deck of a boat being towed with a nylon towing line will receive a far more serious injury. Vision-threatening blunt ocular injuries include the following.

• *Iridodialysis.* The *iris* (the colored portion of the eye) rips at its base, and the pupil becomes D-shaped. You'll also see a black half-moon shape at the periphery of the victim's iris.

• *Traumatic iritis.* A blow to the eyeball causes intense inflammation of the iris and spasm of the structures that control pupil size. The victim complains of deep, aching pain in the eye and sensitivity to light. The eye is diffusely red, the pupil is constricted, and you'll see a red band on the periphery of the victim's cornea.

• *Corneal laceration.* This injury may be hard to see; it can cause a teardrop-shaped pupil and flattening of the front chamber of the eye as fluid leaks out of the wound.

• *Hyphema, or bleeding into the front chamber of the eye.* If you shine a light into the victim's eye, you'll see a collection of blood in the bottom part of the front chamber. Hyphemas can lead to glaucoma and blood staining of the cornea.

• *Detached retina.* A violent blow to the eye can tear the retina, the inner lining of the back chamber of the eye. Fluid from the chamber then leaks behind the retina and detaches it from the back of the eye. Retinal detachment is painless, but the victim will describe a curtain or veil moving across the visual field of his injured eye as the detachment progresses.

• *Dislocated lens.* If the lens is *subluxated* (partially dislocated), the victim will have blurred or double vision in the injured eye. If the lens is dislocated, he'll see only lights and shadows with the affected eye. If the victim's lens is dislocated into the front chamber, you'll be able to see it. If it is pushed into the back chamber, the iris will tremble with head or eye movement.

• *Ruptured globe.* A ruptured eyeball may not be obvious, but the victim complains of sudden impairment of his vision, and you'll notice that the eyeball is soft and the cornea is folded.

• *Foreign object in the eye.* A small fragment of steel can penetrate the eyeball while the victim is using a power tool or hammering on a fitting. He may have no symptoms for a day or so, and then develop decreased vision and dull, poorly localized pain in the eye. If you look carefully, you may find a minute wound in the eyelid, cornea, or sclera.

Treatment

All of these injuries require emergency evaluation by an ophthalmologist. While you are returning to shore, protect the affected eye by taping a paper cup over it. If the victim has a hyphema, have him lie on his back with his head elevated 30 to 45 degrees. If he has a retinal detachment, keep him flat on his back.

Here is a list of "don'ts."

• Don't manipulate the eyeball or the surrounding tissues.
• Don't attempt to remove an impaling object from the globe.
• Don't apply ointments or drops of any kind.
• Don't apply a soft eye patch. (The pressure of the patch may aggravate the injury.)
• Don't let the patient eat or drink anything. (A full stomach will delay emergency surgery.)

•
•
•
•
•

4

CHEST AND ABDOMINAL INJURIES

A gust that he estimated at seventy knots in strength knocked the big sloop over on her side and, he said later, "a wave that was solid green water at least six feet above the deck picked five guys up and threw them at me." Kilroy was pinned against a winch. First thought to be broken ribs, the injury was eventually diagnosed as a ruptured chest cartilage. . . .

—John Rousmaniere, *Fastnet, Force 10*

CHEST INJURIES

Chest injuries are dangerous and hurt like the devil. A cracked rib or separated rib cartilage will present enormous difficulties for you if you are short-crewed. A *pneumothorax* (collapsed lung) might kill you if it's not treated expeditiously. And any injury to the lower chest can be complicated by a life-threatening abdominal injury.

The Chest Bellows

The chest is a bellows. Each time you take a breath, your diaphragm (the bell-shaped muscle which separates the chest and abdominal cavities) pulls down on the lower part of your chest cavity. This expands the chest and creates a relative vacuum which draws air through the respiratory tree and into the lungs. After a second or two, the diaphragm relaxes, the chest cavity contracts, and the lungs recoil and deflate.

Evaluating Chest Wounds

You'll have to rely on your eyes, ears, and fingertips to diagnose serious chest injuries at sea. Sit or lay your patient down in a quiet, well-lighted place, and have him strip to his skivvies. Then examine his chest as follows.

Inspect

Make sure his airway is clear and that he is breathing. Measure his respiratory rate (number of breaths per minute) and note his breathing pattern. The normal respiratory rate at rest is 12 to 20 breaths a minute. Check his color. His skin should be slightly pinkish. If his lips, ears, and fingertips are blue, he is in shock or respiratory distress.

Are his neck veins bulging? Is his trachea (windpipe) deviated to one side? These are both signs of tension pneumothorax (see below).

Do you see any abrasions, lacerations, puncture wounds, or asymmetrical movement?

Feel

Run your hands over the entire chest cage—front and back. Check for tenderness, abnormal movement, or crepitus (grating). Tenderness and crepitus are reliable signs of rib fracture. A bubbly feeling under the skin is caused by air that has escaped from a punctured lung.

Percuss

Tap on the chest with the ends of your long and index fingers. You should hear a slightly hollow sound from the collarbones to about the sixth rib in the front, and from the shoulder blades to about the tenth ribs in the back.

Listen

Listen to the chest with a stethoscope or your bare ear while the victim takes a few deep breaths. If the upper airway is obstructed, you will hear loud, harsh breath sounds. A rattling sound is caused by blood or fluid in the airways. If you hear no breath sounds on one side, and that side also has a hollow sound when you tap on it, the victim probably has a pneumothorax. If the chest sounds dull when you tap on it, he probably has a hemothorax (see pages 59–60).

BLUNT CHEST INJURIES

Rib Fractures

Winches, vents, bitts, cleats, and windlasses are not rib-friendly. If you land chest-first on one of these deck protuberances, you are going to bruise or crack one or more ribs. It's hard to distinguish between these injuries. They both cause intense pain that worsens with deep inspiration and trunk movement. If the victim has tenderness and crepitus over the injured area, and the pain is aggravated when you press on his breastbone when he is supine, you can be sure that he has at least one fractured rib.

Treatment
A 6-inch elastic bandage wrapped around the chest at the level of the injured rib will relieve pain by stabilizing the fracture. An ice pack and analgesics will help, too.

Warning. Fractures of the lower ribs are sometimes associated with liver or spleen injuries. Examine the abdomen carefully, and keep a close eye on your patient's vital signs and skin color. If he has abdominal pain or tenderness, or signs of shock, get on the radio and request immediate evacuation.

Separated Cartilage

In the front of the chest, the ribs are connected to the breastbone by bars of cartilage. A hard fall onto the front of the chest can disrupt the rib-cartilage junction, producing a separated cartilage. These injuries cause a snapping sensation on deep inspiration and take weeks to heal, but are otherwise indistinguishable from fractured ribs.

Treatment
Treatment is the same as for fractured ribs.

Fractured Breastbone

Tremendous force is required to fracture the breastbone, but such forces are not uncommon at sea. Suspect this injury if the victim is slammed into a blunt object and complains of pain in the center of the chest with deep inspiration. He'll have tenderness and crepitus over the breastbone, and the chest may appear to be indented. Complications include heart contusion and lung injury.

Treatment
Prop him up so that he can breathe better, attend to any other injuries, and arrange medical evacuation.

Flail Chest

A "flail chest" is an unstable segment of the chest cage resulting from two or more fractures in each of three or more consecutive ribs. The flail segment moves paradoxically with each breath; i.e., it sinks in when the chest is expanding with inspiration, and pushes out when the chest is contracting with expiration. This hinders the normal flow of air into and out of the lungs, and the underlying lung is usually contused. The flail-chest victim may have no complaint, other than pain, for a day or two. But then he'll develop progressively worsening shortness of breath and respiratory failure.

Treatment
Get the victim to a hospital as quickly as possible.

Pneumothorax (Collapsed Lung)

If a broken rib punctures a lung, air will flow out of the lung and into the chest cavity until the pressure in the chest cavity causes the lung to collapse. The signs and symptoms of a pneumothorax include pain, shortness of breath, diminished breath sounds on the affected side, and a hollow sound when you tap over the affected side of the chest.

Treatment

The victim needs to have a tube inserted into his chest to drain air from the chest cavity and reinflate the lung. Sit him up and make him as comfortable as possible while awaiting evacuation.

Tension Pneumothorax

If a rib creates a one-way valve (flutter valve) when it punctures the surface of the lung, air will be able to flow only one way: out of the lung into the chest cavity. This leads to a *tension pneumothorax*. The chest cavity fills up with air under tremendous tension and pushes the heart, great vessels, and trachea over to the opposite side of the chest, compressing the uninjured lung. Kinks in the great veins prevent the return of venous blood to the heart, and the circulation collapses. The victim turns blue, his neck veins bulge, and he becomes extremely agitated and short of breath. He will die if his chest isn't decompressed immediately.

Treatment

Quickly clean the skin with antiseptic solution and insert the largest intravenous sterile needle you have into the space between the second and third ribs just lateral to the nipple. Guide the needle over the top of the third rib and then straight into the chest until you hear a gush of air as the needle enters the chest cavity. The victim's color and overall appearance will improve dramatically after this life-saving procedure. Leave the needle in place and arrange for emergency evacuation to a hospital.

Hemothorax

A severe blow to the chest, the kind you'd get tumbling down an open hatch or falling out of a bosun's chair, can cause an accumulation of blood in the chest cavity, or *hemothorax*. Usually a complication of rib fractures, a small hemothorax isn't a life-threatening injury, but a large one is. The victim will be anxious, in pain, pale, sweaty, and short of breath. His pulse will be rapid, and his blood pressure low. His chest will sound dull when you percuss the injured side, and you won't hear much air moving into that lung.

Treatment
Make your patient as comfortable as possible while awaiting evacuation to a hospital where the hemothorax can be drained.

PENETRATING CHEST INJURIES

Penetrating chest trauma was one of Captain Joshua Slocum's concerns when he navigated his sloop *Spray* through the Strait of Magellan in 1896. But the aborigines of Tierra del Fuego no longer hail passing mariners with barrages of spears and arrows, and penetrating chest wounds are now uncommon on shipboard.

One form of penetrating chest trauma that you should be familiar with, though, is the *sucking chest wound* (see Figure 13). This can result from a spear-gun injury, a fall onto the pointed end of a boat hook or some other sharp object, or a swordfish attack. If the diameter of the wound approaches the diameter of the windpipe, air will be sucked through the wound into the chest cavity each time the victim takes a breath, and the lung will collapse. Very little air will flow through the windpipe, and he will die of respiratory failure if the problem isn't corrected fast.

Treatment
Cover the wound with any clean bandage within reach: a towel, a sail bag, or even your hand. Once the victim is stabilized, apply a sterile, petrolatum gauze dressing to the wound, and cover it with a sterile 4″ x 4″ gauze pad. Tape the pad on three sides so that air can escape but not enter through the wound. (*Warning:* Don't seal the bandage tight. That will create a tension pneumothorax.) Then, get on the horn and arrange for evacuation.

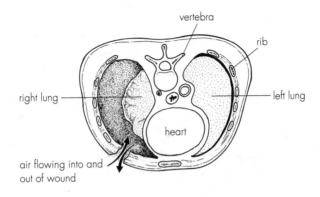

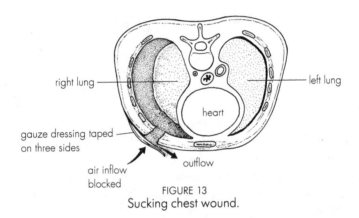

FIGURE 13
Sucking chest wound.

ABDOMINAL INJURIES

If a foaming greyback comes crashing over the stern and slams you belly-down onto a winch or vent, you stand a good chance of lacerating or rupturing your spleen or liver. Such injuries can lead to hemorrhagic shock and death if not diagnosed and treated in a timely fashion. But diagnosis can be tricky. You can lose a lot of blood before the abdomen starts to stretch, and by then it may be too late.

The key to diagnosing these injuries is vigilance. Anyone who sustains a hard blow to the abdomen or lower ribs should be examined carefully and repeatedly. Be on the lookout for early signs of shock: lightheadedness and weakness when the victim sits up; thirst; cool, damp skin; and rapid (110 to 120 beats per minute) pulse. Expose his chest and abdomen and look for bruises, discoloration, or swelling. Warm your hands and feel his belly. Is it soft or rigid? Gently probe under the rib cage with your fingertips. Is there a tender area on either his right (liver) or left (spleen)? Now press over the rest of the abdomen. Localized tenderness and rigidity may be due to a bruise of the abdominal wall, but diffuse rigidity and tenderness, along with signs of early shock, indicate blunt injury to the abdominal organ.

Treatment
Place the victim in the shock position, cover him with blankets, and give him fluids by mouth as desired *(ad lib)*. If you can, start an intravenous line with a large-bore (16 or 18 gauge) catheter and infuse Ringer's lactate as rapidly as possible. While you are tending to your patient, have someone else arrange for emergency evacuation, by helicopter if possible.

Kidney Injuries

A hard fall or a whack in the back or flank by a flying boom or spinnaker pole can injure a kidney. The victim will have pain in the back or the flank, and his urine may be pink-tinged or grossly bloody *(hematuria)*. If the kidney is merely contused, the hematuria will stop after a few hours. If he has substantial pain, feels weak, and continues to pass blood, he may have lacerated or ruptured a kidney.

Treatment
Same as for other abdominal injuries (see above).

.
.
.
.
.

5

FRACTURES AND
DISLOCATIONS

*. . . the captain made a leap for the weather shrouds to get
firm grip and not be washed away . . . but the sea and the
ship's tremendous roll to leeward spun him over end for end
—pitched him a somersault, still clinging to the lines. His
head struck the steel bar at the foot of the shrouds . . . and
cleft it open about a foot. A kneecap was knocked adrift,
and he had other injuries. There he was, a dreadful sight,
flung on his beam ends, blood gushing from his wounded
head . . . a collarbone broken, unable to stand because of
the leg injury, loss of breath, and a bellyful of sea water.
. . . Captain Miethe allowed himself to be helped to the little
hospital down below.*

*Here he took command. The collarbone was no problem.
The mate knew how to strap his shoulder up so that would
mend.*

*"Knock it back," he gave instructions for the shifted
kneecap to be given a suitable tap with a wooden belaying
pin. As for the broken head, it was only skin and such: there
was no fracture of that hard headpiece.*

—Captain Alan Villiers, *War with Cape Horn*

You don't need a belaying pin to treat fractures and dislocations
at sea, but you do need some splinting materials and a little know-
how. You shouldn't get into trouble if you remember that *a fracture
is a soft tissue injury complicated by a broken bone.* Generally, the
safest approach to any fracture or dislocation on shipboard is to
immobilize the injury in a splint until it can be tended by a physician. As long as the skin over the fracture site or dislocated joint
is intact, and there is no sign of compromised circulation or nerve
damage, manipulation of the injury can be delayed for a few hours.
However, if you're in the southern Indian Ocean when your ship-

mate trips over the spinnaker pole and sustains a fracture-dislocation of the ankle, you may have to take a more active role. If his foot turns numb and pale, you'll have to quickly reduce the ankle and restore circulation to his foot.

A SYSTEMATIC APPROACH TO SKELETAL INJURIES

1. *Check the CMS.* CMS refers to Circulation, Motor function, and Sensation. Numbness, weakness, or diminished circulation in the extremity distal to (beyond) the fracture or dislocation means that displaced bone or fracture fragments are stretching or pressing on vessels or nerves. The victim may lose his hand or foot if you don't recognize the problem and do something about it. Here's how to check the CMS.

a. Circulation. Check the pulse at the wrist (just above the thumb side of the hand) or at the ankle (behind the inner knob), as appropriate. Then check the warmth and color of the fingers and toes. If they are cool compared to the uninjured side, and blue or pale instead of pink, the circulation is impaired.

b. Motion. Ask the victim to move the joints below the injury.

c. Sensation. Check for pain sensation by gently pinching the skin below the injury.

2. *Distinguish between bony injury and sprains or bruises.* You will have to make an educated guess as to whether the injury is a fracture or dislocation or just a contusion or sprain. If the limb is grossly deformed, and bone is protruding through the skin, all doubt as to the true nature of the injury will flee your mind. If it isn't deformed, ask the victim to move the extremity. If he can move it through a normal range of motion, it's probably not fractured, and definitely isn't dislocated. Next, gently press on the bone, starting a few inches from the injured area. If it is fractured, it will be quite tender, and you'll feel crepitus, a grinding sensation caused by the bone ends rubbing together. (You also may hear some language that would make Blackbeard the Pirate blush.)

3. *Inspect the skin.* Check the skin over the fracture site. If bone is visible through an open wound, the victim has an *open fracture*. Open fractures are *orthopedic emergencies*. They are virtually always contaminated with bacteria and may be complicated by wound infection or osteomyelitis (bone infection).

Reducing Fractures

If the injured limb is not deformed, it doesn't need to be reduced ("set"). Just "splint 'em as they lie." If the limb *is* deformed, however, the fracture is either *displaced* (the ends are overriding or one fragment is rotated), *angulated,* or both. Angulated or displaced fractures need to be reduced to bring the fragments back into proper position and alignment. Reduction of a displaced fracture will:

1. Relieve stretching and pressure on nerves and blood vessels near the fracture.
2. Reduce bleeding at the fracture site.
3. Prevent a closed fracture from becoming an open fracture.
4. Relieve pain.
5. Enable you to splint the fracture.

Open Fractures

Open fractures are at high risk for infection and must be tended to immediately. First, cover the wound with 4″ x 4″ gauze pads soaked in antiseptic solution, and clean the skin around the wound with antiseptic solution. Then, reduce the fracture by applying longitudinal traction to the limb. Cover the wound with a bulky dressing, and immobilize the limb in a splint. Administer cefadroxil, 1 g stat (immediately), and 500 mg every 12 hours, and arrange for evacuation.

When to Evacuate

Ideally, an uncomplicated fracture or dislocation should be reduced as soon as possible. Open fractures or dislocations and fractures associated with major burns, significant blood loss, spinal-cord injury, nerve damage, or circulatory embarrassment require emergency evacuation to a shoreside hospital.

Splints

You'd be wise to keep an assortment of air splints, padded aluminum splints, wire splints, and SAM splints on board, but you can improvise in an emergency. Oars, paddles, gaffs, fishing rods, newspapers, magazines, charts, sleeping pads, and other shipboard items all make good splints.

Keep these splinting principles in mind when you immobilize a fracture.

1. The splint should immobilize the joints above and below the fracture.

2. Apply longitudinal traction to a fractured limb before applying a splint, but splint dislocated limbs in the position in which you find them.

3. The splint should be well padded, especially over the knees, ankles, elbows, and other bony prominences.

4. The splint should provide some compression over the fracture site but should never be so tight as to impair the circulation. Avoid overinflating air splints. Loosen the distal portion of the splint every two hours to check CMS.

5. Remember the RICE: Rest, Ice, Compression, and Elevation.

UPPER-EXTREMITY FRACTURES

Collarbone

Fractured collarbones are hard to miss. They usually result from a fall onto the side of the shoulder, or a blow on the end of the collarbone from above downward, (e.g., a falling spinnaker pole), and cause swelling, crepitus, deformity, and pain on elevation of the arm.

Treatment
Simply keep the arm in a sling until the victim can move the arm comfortably (7 to 10 days).

Shoulder

A fall onto the shoulder may fracture the upper-arm bone (humerus). You'll note massive swelling just below the shoulder, and the victim won't be able to use his arm.

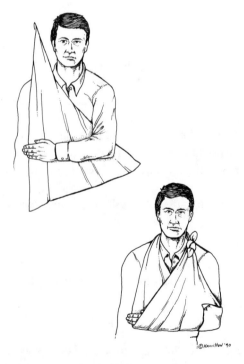

FIGURE 14
Making a sling.

Treatment

Put the injured arm into a sling fashioned out of a triangular bandage, and strap the sling to the body with a leather belt, a 6-inch elastic bandage, or a piece of cloth (see Figure 14). Or simply secure his sleeve to the chest of his shirt with safety pins.

Upper Arm

Fractures of the upper arm (mid-humerus) are unstable and always deformed, characteristically bowing forward at the fracture site. The victim may have a "wrist drop," i.e., inability to extend the wrist or fingers, due to nerve damage.

Treatment

Secure splints to both the inner and outer sides of the upper arm with an elastic bandage, and then put the arm in a sling and *swathe* (band). If there is a wrist drop, apply a "cock-up splint" (see "Wrist" on page 70).

Elbow

If you slip on a wet deck and land with all your weight on your elbow, it will crack.

Treatment

Put the arm in a sling.

Forearm

Either or both forearm bones (ulna and radius) may fracture following a direct blow to the area (e.g., a heavy block falling onto the arm).

Treatment

If the forearm is deformed and CMS is impaired, grasp the arm by the wrist and apply steady, gentle traction. When it looks straight, and you can feel a strong pulse at the wrist, splint it and put the arm in a sling with the elbow flexed to 90 degrees.

Wrist

A fall on the outstretched hand may either sprain or fracture the wrist. If the injured wrist is bent like a fork, it's fractured. But the absence of deformity doesn't mean that it's not fractured.

Treatment
Immobilize the wrist in a cock-up splint in a position of function. Have your patient hold a balled-up pair of socks in the palm of his hand. Place the wrist and hand on a firm, 10-inch-long splint. Then wrap a 3-inch elastic bandage around the hand from the knuckles to the upper forearm, and put the arm in a sling.

If the fingers are cold and blue, and there is no pulse at the wrist, the injury may be a fracture-dislocation. Grasp the victim's hand with yours as though you were going to shake hands and pull straight out until the deformity is corrected. If color and warmth return to the hand, apply a cock-up splint.

Hand and Fingers

If you think the victim has fractured a *metacarpal* (long bone of the hand), apply a cock-up splint.

Finger Fracture
Fingers consist of three long bones, called the *proximal* (closest to the hand), *middle,* and *distant phalanges.* They are frequently fractured on shipboard.

Treatment
Reduce a fracture of the proximal or middle phalanx by pulling straight out on the finger until it looks straight. Then, with the finger in the "James position" (the finger flexed 70 to 90 degrees at the knuckle, the first finger joint flexed 15 to 20 degrees, and the second finger joint flexed 5 to 10 degrees), apply an aluminum

splint to the palm side of the digit from fingertip to the base of the hand. A simpler solution is to simply tape the finger to the adjoining finger ("buddy taping") and encourage your patient to use the finger as normally as possible while the fracture heals.

Mallet Finger

If a whisker pole or some other hard object strikes the tip of your finger and snaps it down, you may get a *mallet* finger. You won't be able to fully extend the tip of the finger because the extensor tendon has been pulled out of its insertion into the base of the distal phalanx.

Treatment

Apply a short splint along the top of the finger over the middle and distal phalanges, with the last joint slightly hyperextended. The tendon will heal in about three weeks.

Crushed Finger Tip

Crushed finger tips should be thoroughly cleaned in antiseptic solution, covered with Adaptic and a sterile gauze dressing, and protected with a short U-shaped splint.

FRACTURES OF THE SPINE

Back

Most shipboard back injuries fall into the category of *lumbar strain*. Any twisting, bending, or lifting movement can stretch or tear the muscles and ligaments of the lower (lumbar) spine and cause terrific pain and stiffness in the small of your back. If you also have severe, electric-shock-like pain running down the back of your leg, you probably have an *intervertebral disk* injury. The best remedy for either condition is a day or two of bed rest, gentle massage, warm compresses, and analgesics.

Falling out of a bosun's chair never hurt anyone, but those hard landings on the deck will get you every time. Such falls can cause *compression fractures* of the vertebral bodies, usually in the midback area, or a *fracture-dislocation* of the spine. The latter is usually associated with signs of spinal-cord injury, such as weakness and loss of feeling below the chest or waist.

Assessment and Treatment

When assisting a crew member who has fallen out of the rigging, first tend to the ABCs. Immobilize his neck if you think it may be injured, and then look for signs of head injury (see Chapter 3). Next, do a quick neurologic exam to rule out spinal cord injury: Have him raise his arms over his head against resistance, and check his grip strength. Then have him flex his hips and knees, and ask him to wiggle his toes. Use a safety pin or toothpick to check for loss of sensation. Starting at his nipples, lightly poke both sides of his chest, both arms and hands, and then both legs and feet. If you find no weakness or numbness, carefully log-roll him onto one side and check for fractures by gently thumping with your fingertips over his spine from neck to tailbone. If you find localized tenderness, assume that there is a fracture at that level. Keep him immobilized, but make him as comfortable as possible while you are returning to shore. Nubaine, 10 mg intramuscularly (IM) may be necessary to control his pain.

Pelvis, Hip, and Thigh

Generally, it takes a tremendous force to fracture one of these large bones. *Fractured femurs* (thigh bones) are usually obvious. The thigh will be swollen, deformed, and very painful, and the victim won't be able to move the injured leg.

Treatment

Have one person grasp the victim's foot and apply steady traction to the leg while another person applies countertraction to the pelvis. When the thigh looks straight, strap an oar, paddle, or spar from armpit to beyond the foot, and a shorter splint to the inner aspect of the thigh from the groin to the foot (see Figure 15). Then put a little padding under the knees to keep them flexed

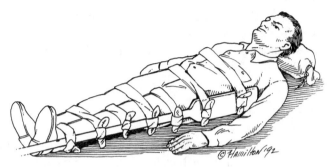

FIGURE 15
Splinting a fractured thigh.

5 to 10 degrees. If you can't find a suitable splint, strap the victim's legs together. Give Vicodin ES, one tablet every 4 to 6 hours as needed, or Nubaine, 10 mg intramuscularly every 4 hours as needed.

Hip fractures cause pain in the hip or groin. Thump the bottom of the victim's heel with your fist. If this produces pain in the groin, he probably has a hip fracture. Pain on movement of the leg and shortening and outward rotation of the leg are also reliable signs of hip fracture.

Treatment
Splint the leg as you would a fractured femur, and give appropriate analgesics.

Check for *pelvic fractures* by putting one hand over each iliac crest (the large bones on each side at waist level) and press inward toward the belly button. If this produces pain in the groin, or if there is tenderness to direct pressure over the iliac crests, groin, or pubic area, he probably has a fractured pelvis. If the victim has only minimal tenderness, and he can walk without much difficulty, he probably has a contusion or a small, stable fracture.

Treatment
If the victim is unable to walk, he may have multiple pelvic fractures. Place some padding between his thighs and under his knees, then bandage his knees and ankles together.

Fractures of the pelvis, hip, and femur can bleed extensively, and are often associated with severe soft tissue injuries and shock. Have a shipmate get on the radio and arrange for medical evacuation while you stabilize the victim.

Kneecap

The kneecap doesn't have much padding and is not hard to fracture. A simple contusion will cause swelling and pain; but if you feel crepitus when you press down on the kneecap, it's probably broken.

Treatment
If there is no deformity, apply a cylindrical splint from groin to ankle and allow the victim to walk as tolerated. If the kneecap is deformed, and the victim cannot extend his knee, it may need to be surgically repaired. Apply a compression dressing (several layers of gauze and ABD pads secured with Kling gauze or an elastic bandage) and head for port.

Lower Leg

If you get thrown across the deck and slammed into the scuppers by several tons of cold, green Atlantic Ocean, you may fracture your tibia (leg bone). Fractures of the upper tibia usually involve the knee joint, which may swell to the size of a mooring buoy. Fractures of the shaft of the tibia are often angulated and open, and the fibula (the thin bone lateral to the tibia) is usually fractured also.

Treatment
Apply traction to the leg by pulling down on the ankle. When it appears straight, splint it. If bone is protruding from a wound, cleanse the wound with antiseptic solution and apply a sterile dressing. Then reduce and splint the fracture. Give Nubaine,

10 mg intramuscularly every 4 hours, as needed to control pain.

Ankle

You can usually distinguish between an ankle sprain and a fracture by pressing over the bony knobs on both sides of the ankle. Tenderness, deformity, and crepitus indicate a fracture. If the foot is discolored and bent at a weird angle, you may be looking at a fracture-dislocation of the ankle.

Treatment
Apply some padding to the ankle and then secure a SAM splint to the bottom of the foot and up the back of the leg to the knee with an elastic bandage. If you don't have a SAM splint, a pillow placed under the ankle and taped across the top will do nicely. If the ankle is dislocated, grasp the foot with the heel in your right (dominant) hand and place your left hand over the top of the foot. Then pull on the foot until the ankle snaps back into place. The victim will feel better immediately, and normal color will return to the foot as the circulation returns.

Foot

If you fall onto the deck while shinnying down the backstay, and land flat on your feet, you'll very likely fracture your heel or the metatarsals (long bones) of your feet. If your back hurts, you may have a compression fracture of the spine also.

Treatment
Apply a cotton cast (a large, soft dressing and elastic bandage) to the heel and keep it elevated and iced. Wear wooden clogs or stiff-soled boots until metatarsal and big-toe fractures heal. (Tape four or five tongue depressors across the sole of the shoe at its widest part to reduce pressure on the fracture.) A fractured toe can be treated by simply inserting a wisp of cotton between the toe and its buddy and taping the two toes together.

DISLOCATIONS

A dislocated joint is an orthopedic emergency. Blood vessels, nerves, muscles, and ligaments are stretched whenever a bone pops out of joint, and the sooner the joint is reduced, the better. If you put it off too long, swelling and muscle spasm will make retrieving a fouled anchor seem simple in comparison.

Treatment

If there is a deep wound over the joint, or bone is protruding, the dislocation is "open." Clean the wound with antiseptic solution and cover it with a sterile bandage before you reduce the dislocation. Administer cefadroxil, 1 g immediately and 500 mg every 12 hours. Remember to check CMS before and after reduction.

Shoulder

The shoulder can be levered out of joint by a backward force against an elevated arm. Don't confuse this injury with a separated shoulder or fracture of the upper humerus. These are the hallmarks of a dislocated shoulder.

1. The shoulder contour is "squared off."
2. The arm is held out from the body.
3. The victim can't place his hand on his uninjured shoulder.

Treatment

Here are two effective reduction techniques.

1. Have the victim lie prone on the cabin top or a dinghy with the injured arm hanging down. Then attach 10 to 15 pounds of weight to his wrist with strips of cloth or gauze (see Figure 16). The shoulder should slip back into joint within fifteen minutes.

2. Position the victim as above and sit or kneel next to him. Pull down on his upper arm until you feel the shoulder slip back into joint.

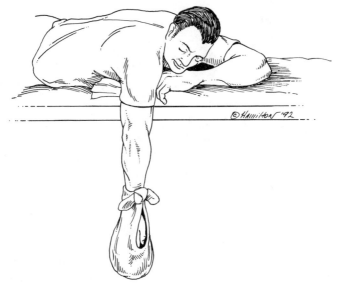

FIGURE 16
Reducing a dislocated shoulder.

You'll know when the shoulder is reduced. Your patient will break out in a beatific smile, and the shoulder will once again have a normal, rounded contour. Keep the arm in a sling for three weeks so that the stretched shoulder capsule can heal.

Separated Shoulder

A separation of the shoulder is a disruption of the A-C (acromioclavicular) joint that joins the end of the collarbone and the shoulder blade (scapula). It results from a fall directly onto the shoulder or a hard blow to the shoulder. In a *partial separation,* the ligaments that support the A-C joint are incompletely torn, and the victim has moderate swelling and tenderness over the end of the collarbone. In a *complete separation,* the ligaments are completely torn, and the end of the collarbone rides high because it is no longer connected to the scapula.

Treatment

Immobilize the shoulder in a sling until the pain and swelling subside. Then have your patient start to use the arm.

Elbow

If a shipmate takes a tumble down the companionway and falls on his arm, the force of the blow may drive the forearm bones backward out of the elbow joint. The elbow will look and feel deformed. (If you feel crepitus, the elbow may be fractured as well as dislocated.)

Treatment

If you are within several hours of medical assistance, and the CMS is good, simply apply ice and put the arm in a sling. However, if you cannot feel a pulse at the wrist and the hand is turning blue, you should attempt to reduce the elbow. Stand in front of the victim and apply steady longitudinal traction on the forearm while a helper exerts countertraction on the upper arm. You'll hear a clunk as the elbow reduces. Apply a compression dressing to the elbow and rest it in a sling for two weeks.

Finger

The first finger joint may be dislocated when the finger is struck or hyperextended by a winch or some other moving object. Dislocated fingers are grossly deformed and easy to diagnose.

Treatment

Pull straight out on the digit with one hand and push against the base of the dislocated bone with the thumb of your other hand until the bone slips back into joint. Then buddy-tape the finger to its partner for 10 days.

Hip

A violent force, such as a fall from the masthead, is required to dislocate a hip, which is a very stable ball-and-socket joint. In an *anterior dislocation*, the thigh is flexed and held out to the side. In a *posterior dislocation*, the leg is shortened and rotated inward.

Treatment

Time is of the essence in hip dislocations. The longer the hip is out of socket, the greater the probability of damage to the sciatic nerve, vascular impairment, and degeneration of the ball part of the joint. Give the victim Nubaine, 10 mg intramuscularly, and then use one of these techniques to reduce his hip.

1. *Allis method.* Place the victim on his back and exert traction on the leg in line with the deformity. Then slowly bend the knee and hip to 90 degrees. Straddle him, place his leg between your thighs, and wrap your hands behind his knee. Then have the biggest crew member press down on his pelvis, while you continue to exert traction on the thigh and gently rotate the leg back and forth until you feel the hip go in.

2. *Stimson method.* Place the patient in a prone position on a table with the hip flexed over the end of the table. With an assistant stabilizing the pelvis by extending the uninjured leg, go through the same maneuvers used in the Allis method, but pull toward the floor.

After you have reduced the hip, confine your patient to bed for 24 hours. Then get him up on crutches. If you can't reduce the hip, splint it in a comfortable position and arrange evacuation.

Kneecap

If you twist your knee while running down a gangplank, you may dislocate your kneecap. A direct blow to the inner side of the kneecap will do the job too. The kneecap will be pushed to the outside, and the knee will be flexed 45 to 60 degrees.

Treatment

The kneecap will pop back into place if you slowly straighten the knee while you press inward on its lateral border. After it's reduced, apply a long splint with the knee fully extended. Walking is permissible.

·
·
·
·
·

6

SHIPBOARD DENTISTRY

*For the Toothach I have found the following medicine very
available, Brimstone and Gunpowder compounded with
butter, rub the mandible with it, the outside being first
warm'd.*

—John Josselyn,
An Account of Two Voyages to New-England

This brimstone-butter-gunpowder compound would probably be
more suitable as a caulking compound than as a toothache remedy.
Fortunately, such concoctions have gone the way of the astrolabe
and the steering oar. Read on for a description of the modern
approach to shipboard dental emergencies.

DENTAL ANATOMY 101

To deal with some of the dental problems you're likely to encounter on a long voyage, you need a working knowledge of dental
anatomy (see Figure 17). Teeth may seem inert, but that's only
because they are covered with a hard layer of *enamel* that covers
the upper portion of a deeper hard layer called the *dentin*. Like all
tissues, teeth are supplied with blood vessels and nerves. They
travel through a central cavity called the *pulp*. The *crown* is the
visible portion of the tooth that extends above the gums (*gingiva*).
The *root* of the tooth tapers and fits into a socket in the *alveolar
bone* of the jaw.

THE SHIPBOARD DENTAL KIT

You won't need a dental chair, Muzak, or one of those fancy water
dispensers to deal with dental problems at sea, but you will need a

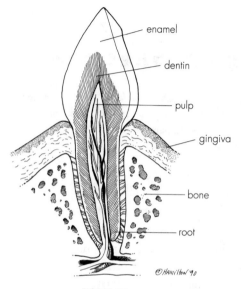

FIGURE 17
Cross-section of a tooth.

few medications and instruments to treat cracked teeth, abscesses, and lost fillings. I recommend that you collect the following items and stow them in a small box in your cabin. You can buy most of these materials at any drugstore. The dental instruments can be purchased at a dental supply store.

- eugenol (oil of cloves)
- vanilla extract
- tea bags
- zinc oxide powder
- cotton pellets
- cotton rolls
- 2" x 2" cotton gauze
- Cavit (premixed filling material)
- IRM (intermediate restorative material)

- Express Putty
- dental mirror
- dental wax
- small cotton pliers
- toothpicks
- electrical tape
- pen light
- dental broach
- Dremel moto-tool 380
- Formocresol

Now that you've mastered dental anatomy and have a dental kit, it's time for you to sink your teeth into the problem of diagnosing and treating some of the common dental emergencies.

TOOTHACHE

Tom Sawyer spent much of his time rafting on the Mississippi, but he turned to his Aunt Polly for help with such things as toothaches:

> *The old lady made one end of the silk thread fast to Tom's tooth with a loop and tied the other to the bedpost. Then she seized the chunk of fire and suddenly thrust it almost to the boy's face. The tooth hung dangling by the bedpost, now.*
>
> —Mark Twain, *The Adventures of Tom Sawyer*

Aunt Polly believed in the radical cure. As the shipboard dentist, you should take a more discerning and analytical approach to the patient with a toothache. Ask him *when* the toothache started, *where* it hurts, and *what* provokes the pain (chewing? hot food? cold food? sweets?). Does he have a steady ache or a throbbing pain? (An ache is often caused by a gingival infection, whereas a throbbing pain usually signifies a problem within the tooth.) Examine his teeth, his gums, and the floor of his mouth. Look for loose, fractured, or decayed teeth; pus; and swelling of the gingiva, inside of the cheek, or floor of the mouth. Check for sensitive teeth by tapping or pressing on the teeth with a tongue blade. Then observe your patient's neck for swelling. Use your fingers to feel under his jaw and the front and back of his neck for swollen, tender lymph nodes. After taking a history and doing a brief examination, you should be able to place his toothache in one of the following categories.

Pulpitis

The pulp that houses the blood vessels and nerve supply to the teeth is prone to inflammation, especially when the tooth becomes decayed or when a filling falls out. Pulpitis causes moderate to severe pain, especially after the tooth is exposed to heat, cold, or sweets, but the toothache may occur spontaneously. The pain is diffuse, and the patient may have difficulty localizing it to either top or bottom. Direct pressure won't help you to identify the offending tooth, but an ice cube or cold food will. Touch the ice to each of the teeth on the painful side of the mouth. A blood-curdling scream indicates that you have found the sore tooth.

Treatment
   1. Use a piece of gauze to dry the tooth.
   2. Remove debris from the pulp cavity with a toothpick or a cotton pellet held with cotton pliers.
   3. Anesthetize the tooth by swabbing with eugenol or vanilla extract.
   4. Mix a small amount of zinc oxide powder with a few drops of eugenol to form a paste, and apply it to the tooth with a toothpick or cotton pliers.
   5. Alternatively, you can use IRM or Cavit to make a filling. Squeeze a little onto your finger, roll it into a small cone, and apply it to the tooth. Have the patient bite it into place. Then shape it with a toothpick. (This temporary filling will wear out after a few days. Put in new fillings as needed.)
   6. Administer Tylenol No. 3, 1 to 2 every 4 hours, or Vicodin ES, 1 every 4 hours, as needed.

Lost Filling

The first sign of a lost filling is sudden sensitivity to hot or cold foods. The patient will notice a sharp edge to his tooth, and complain of pain on chewing. The defect in the tooth is usually quite obvious to both the patient and the examiner.

Treatment
   1. Remove food debris and dry the tooth with cotton gauze.
   2. If necessary, anesthetize the tooth with eugenol and vanilla extract.

3. Make a soft mix of IRM or Cavit and place it into the tooth. Have the patient mold the material by biting down and chewing on it.

4. Wipe off the excess material.

Periapical Periodontitis

Periodontitis is analogous to a joint sprain. It's caused by inflammation of the supporting structures at the base of a tooth and causes a constant throbbing pain. The tooth is sensitive to direct pressure, but there is no gingival swelling, as there would be if the tooth were infected.

Periapical periodontitis can be caused by trauma, e.g., biting an uncooked popcorn kernel or sustaining a direct blow from a swinging boom or flying debris during a gale. It may also be secondary to leakage of necrotic material from decaying pulp. The tooth is extruded (pushed out) slightly, so chewing is painful.

Treatment

1. Place a wad of gauze on the nonaffected side to take some of the pressure off the affected tooth.

2. Give analgesics as needed.

3. Keep the patient on a soft diet until the inflammation subsides.

Myofascial Pain-Dysfunction (MPD) Syndrome

Every sailor knows stress. It's that cramp that grabs the back of your neck as you try to move off a lee shore against a powerful current and an onshore breeze, or the jaw-clenching tension you feel when you enter an unmarked channel on a moonless night. Ulysses had some tense moments as his galley ran the gauntlet between Scylla and Charybdis:

> Then we entered the Straits in great fear of mind, for on the
> one hand was Scylla, and on the other dread Charybdis kept
> sucking up the salt water. As she vomited it up, it was like

> the water in a cauldron when it is boiling over upon a great
> fire, and the spray reached the top of the rocks on either side.
> When she began to suck again, we could see the water all
> inside whirling round and round, and it made a deafening
> sound as it broke against the rocks . . . the men were at
> their wits' ends for fear. While we were taken up with this
> and expected each moment to be our last, Scylla pounced
> down suddenly upon us and snatched six of my best men. I
> was looking at once after both ship and men, and in a
> moment I saw their hands and feet ever so high above me,
> struggling in the air as Scylla was carrying them off, and I
> heard them call out my name in one last despairing cry. . . .
> Even so did Scylla land these panting creatures on her rock
> and munch them up at the mouth of her den, while they
> screamed and stretched out their hands to me in their mortal
> agony.
>
> —Homer, *The Odyssey*

Stress-induced muscle tension triggers spasm of the muscles in the back of the neck and the muscles of mastication around the jaw. The painful spasms cause more stress, then more muscle tension, and so on, in a vicious cycle. MPD causes pain in front of the ear, headache, and painful chewing.

Treatment
1. Soft diet.
2. Warm compresses.
3. Ibuprofen, 400 to 600 mg four times a day.

INFECTIONS

Acute Apical Abscess

If a cavity is ignored long enough, bacteria will spread into the pulp, and from there into the tooth socket. An apical abscess causes a throbbing toothache or generalized aching in several teeth. You can identify the infected tooth by tapping on the tooth, by having the patient bite down on a Q-tip cotton swab, or by applying ice to it. You'll see some swelling around the root of the tooth and on the cheek side of the jaw. The swelling may extend under the jaw and into the deep neck spaces. This swelling can cause difficulty opening the jaw and can compromise the airway.

Treatment

1. Use the Dremel moto-tool to drill a hole into the top or side of the tooth to drain the pus.

2. Use a broach to remove as much of the pulp as you can.

3. Soak a small cotton pellet with Formocresol and put it into the drill hole.

4. Administer penicillin VK, 500 mg four times a day for 10 days.

5. Apply warm compresses to the cheek.

6. Keep the patient on a soft diet, and give him appropriate analgesics.

Periodontal Abscess (Gum Abscess)

When food particles get trapped between the tooth and gum, a periodontal abscess can form. The gum becomes swollen and tender, but the tooth will not be sensitive to pressure.

Treatment

1. Anesthetize the affected area with eugenol or vanilla extract.

2. Probe under the gum line with a split tongue blade to drain the abscess and remove food particles. (Or, use a scalpel to incise the gingiva and drain the pus.)

3. Administer tetracycline, 500 mg four times a day for 10 days if your patient has a fever.

4. Have the patient floss twice a day and rinse his mouth frequently with warm salt water.

Pericoronitis

Pericoronitis is marked by redness, swelling, and tenderness of the gingiva over an unerupted wisdom tooth. Repeated biting traumatizes the thin layer of gingiva covering the tooth and leads to infection. The patient complains of a sore throat and pain on opening his mouth.

Treatment
 1. Numb the gingiva with eugenol or vanilla extract.
 2. Excise the flap with a #11 scalpel.
 3. Have the patient bite on gauze or on a wet tea bag for a few minutes to control bleeding.
 3. Administer penicillin VK, 500 mg every 6 hours for 10 days if your patient has a fever and swollen lymph glands in the neck.
 4. Have him rinse his mouth with warm salt water four times a day.

DENTAL TRAUMA

Fractured Tooth

A fractured tooth will be obvious if a sizable fragment is chipped off. The tooth will survive if the fracture doesn't extend through the dentin into the pulp cavity. If you see bleeding from the center of the tooth, the vital structures in the pulp cavity have been exposed and the tooth is doomed if you don't get to a dentist within 48 hours. You can localize a hairline fracture by having the patient bite on a rubber eraser or Q-tip. Then place a pen light against the involved tooth and look for fracture lines.

Treatment
 1. Numb the tooth with eugenol or vanilla extract.
 2. Remove the loose fragment with forceps.

3. If the pulp cavity is exposed, use a dental broach to extirpate the pulp tissue.

4. Soak a cotton pellet with Formocresol and plug the opening in the pulp cavity to keep food out, or

5. Cap the tooth with IRM or Cavit.

6. See a dentist within 5 to 10 days.

Loose Teeth

You should make every attempt to salvage loose and avulsed teeth. Most loose teeth will do fine if they are in good position or pushed in a little. If the tooth is crooked or partially out of the socket, reposition it with your fingers. Then mix up a batch of Express Putty and mold the material over the loose tooth and two adjoining teeth on each side. Or use dental wax to splint the tooth.

A completely avulsed tooth can be salvaged if you replace it immediately. Hold it by the crown and rinse it off in saline solution or the cleanest water available, then put it back into the socket. Apply a dental wax splint and administer penicillin VK, 250 mg every 6 hours for 7 days.

Lost Crown

Apply a few drops of eugenol to the tooth. Then rinse the crown in water or saline solution and place it back on the tooth. When you are satisfied with the fit, remove the crown, apply a few drops of Cavit, and reposition it on the tooth. Have the victim bite down on the crown until it settles into place. Remove the excess Cavit with a toothpick.

Broken Denture

Wash and dry the denture, then repair it with strips of electrical tape along the tongue sides. Use a dental adhesive to secure it in the mouth. If you have epoxy glue on board, mix up a batch and glue the broken surfaces together. But make certain you get a precise fit, or the denture will be too uncomfortable to use. (Don't use a rapid-setting glue to repair a broken denture. It will set too fast to assure precise alignment of the edges of the denture.)

REMEMBER: You can avoid many dental emergencies by visiting your dentist for a dental overhaul before setting out on a long voyage.

•
•
•
•
•

7

SHIPBOARD DERMATOLOGY

On old-time sailors it was fashionable to tattoo a pig on one foot and a rooster on the other. An old-time bos'n claimed that anyone so marked could not drown, for these creatures despised the water.

—Horace Beck, *Folklore and the Sea*

Have you ever wondered why fish have scales or why sharks have such thick, tough hides? If they had skin like ours instead of their armorlike integument, fish wouldn't survive long in an environment teeming with skin-tunneling parasites, spiculed sponges, razor-sharp coral, fanged bristle worms, and virulent, skin-invading bacteria. These submarine hazards can make life miserable for swimmers and divers. If you don't want them to get under your skin, read on.

SPONGE DERMATITIS

Sponges are invertebrate animals that attach to coral beds or to rocks on the sea floor. Their tough but elastic skeletons contain sharp spicules of silica or calcium carbonate which can inflict painful cuts and abrasions on unwary divers. And sponges play host to a bewildering array of coelenterates, crustaceans, echinoderms, annelid worms, hydrozoans, mollusks, algae, and fish (see Chapter 17) which can cause "sponge diver's disease." Many sponges produce skin irritants known as *crinotoxins*.

Sponges cause two forms of dermatitis.

1. *An itchy, poison-ivy-like rash.* Common sponge offenders include the Hawaiian or West Indies fire sponge (Hawaiian Islands and Florida Keys), the "poison bun sponge," and the red moss sponge, a native of Northeast coastal waters. Within a few hours after skin contact with one of these sponges, you'll develop itching, burning, local joint swelling, stiffness, and blistering. Usually only the hand is affected, but if a large skin area is involved, you may develop fever, chills, dizziness, malaise, and cramps. Mild reactions subside spontaneously within a few days.

2. *An irritant dermatitis.* This condition results from penetration of the skin by calcium carbonate or silica spicules. Crinotoxins may enter the skin through puncture wounds created by these spicules and cause your skin to peel days to months later.

Treatment

It's difficult to tell which of these two forms of sponge dermatitis you are dealing with, so follow this combined treatment plan.

1. Dry the skin gently with a towel.

2. Remove the spicules with adhesive tape or a facial peel.

3. Apply diluted (5%) vinegar soaks three times a day for 20 to 30 minutes. (You can use isopropyl alcohol if you don't have vinegar.)

4. Coat the affected area with a moisturizing cream (Neutrogena, Vaseline Intensive Care, Eucerin, etc.) thrice daily.

5. Apply hydrocortisone 1% ointment twice a day if the area is itchy or intensely inflamed. If weeping blisters and crusty inflammation develop, you may need to give prednisone according to this tapered schedule: 60 mg a day for 4 days; then 40 mg a day for 3 days; then 20 mg a day for 3 days; and finally 10 mg a day for 2 days.

6. Control intense itching with diphenhydramine, 25 to 50 mg every 6 hours as needed.

7. Watch for signs of infection.

"Sponge diver's disease" is treated like any coelenterate poisoning (see Chapter 17).

Prevention

Wear gloves when handling sponges, especially if you intend to break them apart.

SEAWEED DERMATITIS

Mariners have cussed seaweed since the first galleons became stranded in the Sargasso Sea. Not only can it foul your rudder or propeller, it can also cause a nasty dermatitis.

North Sea fishermen get a poison-ivy-like rash called the "Dogger Bank itch" when they handle mats of sea moss containing seachervil that are caught in their nets. The rash may disappear quickly, or the exposed skin may swell and break out in blisters. It's treated with Burow's solution compresses, calamine lotion, and antihistamines.

Seaweed dermatitis is usually caused by *algae*, plants which have no true roots, stems, or leaves, and which range in size from microscopic (diatoms) to over 300 feet (kelp). *Microcoleus* is an olive- to dark-green stinging seaweed that grows in mats throughout the Caribbean Sea and the Pacific and Indian oceans. It causes outbreaks of seaweed dermatitis from March to September in Florida coastal waters, and from June through September in the Hawaiian Islands. (Freshwater blue-green algae can also cause dermatitis.) Several minutes to hours after leaving the water, you may develop a burning, red, itchy rash under your bathing suit. Later, the skin blisters and peels.

Treatment
Thoroughly wash the affected area with warm soap and water, rinse with isopropyl alcohol, and apply 1% hydrocortisone ointment twice daily. You can *prevent* seaweed dermatitis by simply showering with soap and water and washing your swimsuit as soon as you exit algae-ridden waters.

SWIMMER'S ITCH

Cercarial dermatitis, a.k.a. "swimmer's itch," "clam digger's itch," and "lakeside disease," is what you get when cercariae (larvae) of a nonhuman-parasitic flatworm confuse you with their normal rodent, bird, or ungulate hosts. These schistosomes ("blood flukes") are found in fresh and salt water throughout the world. Swimmer's itch is the bane of swimmers and divers in most American coastal waters and in many freshwater lakes in the upper Midwest. You're especially likely to contract swimmer's itch during warm weather, when there is a strong onshore wind, when there is seaweed in the surf, and where there is a great deal of submerged vegetation.

Swimmer's itch starts shortly after you emerge from cercariae-infested waters. When your skin dries, cercariae attempt to bore through it and into your veins, but they are unable to penetrate the deep layer of the skin. Your immune system reacts to the invaders with an inflammatory response which walls them off and destroys them.

The first symptom of swimmer's itch is a prickling sensation, followed a few minutes to an hour later by hives. The hives evolve into flat red lesions and then into intensely itchy papules, or bumps. Small blisters and pustules may form a couple of days later. The rash mainly involves exposed skin, is incredibly itchy for the first 3 days, and then slowly resolves over 7 to 14 days. Excessive scratching may cause excoriations, pustules, scabs, and secondary infection.

Treatment

You can control mild itching by applying a 50:50 solution of isopropyl alcohol and calamine lotion as needed. Diphenhydramine in the usual dosages will help also. If the itching is severe, take a tapered course of prednisone as described for sponge dermatitis.

Prevention

Grab a dry towel as soon as you get out of the water and vigorously dry yourself off before the little monsters start burrowing into your skin.

SEABATHERS' ERUPTION

"Seabathers' eruption" is a mystery malady. Its cause is unknown, but its symptoms are similar to those of seaweed dermatitis and swimmer's itch. It begins, a few hours after swimming in ocean water, with red, itchy wheals or papules in areas covered by your swimsuit. After 2 or 3 days, the rash disappears. You can control the itching by applying calamine lotion containing 1% menthol. You can *prevent* seabathers' eruption by washing with soap and water immediately after getting out of the water.

MARINE WORMS

It seems as though every form of life in the sea is endowed with sharp teeth, tentacles, claws, or poison with which to defend itself or kill prey. The marine annelid (segmented) worms are no exception. There are over six thousand species of these worms swimming about the oceans of the world or groping about on the sea floor. Some are toxic, some have teeth, and they all are armed with rows of sharp *setae* (bristles) that can puncture skin.

If you think night crawlers are big, you've never seen a bristle worm. These monsters grow to be 12 inches in length and one inch thick, and are found just about everywhere. In Caribbean and Florida waters they hang out on the bottom under rocks, in sponges, and on coral. When a diver handles the worm, its body contracts and its bristles become erect. They puncture the diver's skin and detach like cactus spines.

Sandworms dwell in huge numbers in coastal sand and mud. They have large, sharp fangs which they extrude to bite prey and human transgressors.

The bites and stings of marine worms cause bee-sting-like pain. The area around the wound becomes red and swollen, but the pain subsides after a few minutes or hours, and the inflammation subsides in a few days.

Treatment

Remove visible bristles with fine tweezers or forceps. Then use adhesive tape or facial peel to remove the finer setae. Finally, sponge the area with vinegar, isopropyl alcohol, or a paste of meat tenderizer.

SEA LOUSE DERMATITIS

The varmints that cause sea louse dermatitis aren't lice at all. They are tiny crustaceans—cousins of crabs, shrimp, and lobsters —that cruise temperate and tropical coastal waters. But they do *bite* like lice, attaching to a swimmer's hand or foot with vice-grip jaws and inflicting a sudden, sharp sting that leaves a pinpoint, bleeding wound.

Treatment

Clean the wound with soap and water, and then apply a coat of antibiotic ointment.

SOAPFISH DERMATITIS

Soapfish should get an award for originality. Can you imagine, in a world inhabited by razor-toothed barracuda and stingrays with poison-tipped barbs in their tails, a fish that kills its enemies by secreting a cloud of "soap"? Well, it works, because the "milk" that the soapfish secretes is lethal to other fish. The mucus won't kill a human, but try to grab the soapfish and you'll get an irritating rash.

Treatment

Wash off the mucus and apply Burow's solution soaks as needed.

SALTWATER BACTERIA

There are three groups of saltwater bacteria that can cause serious skin infections.

Mycobacterium marinum

This bacterium is a saltwater cousin of the bacillus that causes tuberculosis. It *won't* give you TB, but it *can* give you a chronic skin infection. It tends to infect only the cool skin of the ends of the extremities and rarely involves lymph nodes. *Mycobacterium*'s modus operandi is to gain entry to the body through a fresh cut or puncture wound, colonize the wound, and produce cellulitis as it spreads through the surrounding skin. If the infection is not recognized and treated, it may spread to local bones and joints, form skin nodules, and cause the skin over the infected area to peel.

Mycobacterium infection may show up as red papules that crop up 3 to 4 weeks after the skin is exposed to *Mycobacterium*. These papules enlarge, harden, and become scaly and ulcerated. They are called *granulomas*, and they appear in lines over the superficial lymph vessels.

Treatment
TMP-SMX or tetracycline may lick *Mycobacterium* skin infections if they are recognized in the early stages, but that's a trick. Without treatment, the nodules and granulomas heal in 2 to 3 years.

Erysipelothrix rhusiopathiae

Erysipelothrix causes *erysipeloid*, or "fish handlers' disease," an infection of the hands and fingers in people who handle live fish, crabs, and shellfish. *Erysipelothrix* bacteria enter abrasions and puncture wounds in the hands, and after a few days cause a painful, itchy, raised violet area. The wound swells and drains pus. A clear, infection-free area develops beyond this swollen purple-red area, and beyond that a well-circumscribed, advancing, red or violet ring. The area is warm and tender, and the infection usually spreads to the adjoining finger and often·up into the wrist and forearm. Satellite infections may form, and you may get a mild fever.

Treatment
Erysipeloid clears spontaneously in 1 to 3 weeks, but you can hasten the healing process by taking penicillin VK, 250 mg every 6 hours, or cefadroxil, 500 mg every 12 hours. Continue the medication for 7 to 10 days.

Vibrio Bacteria

It is only fitting that sharks, the most dangerous *fish* in the sea, should harbor in their mouths the most dangerous marine *bacteria.* If a shark's bite doesn't kill you, a *Vibrio* wound infection just might. And almost any wound sustained in salt water can become infected with *vibrio* bacteria, which are found in shallow and estuarine waters throughout the temperate zone. *Vibrio* can also cause gastroenteritis and ear and sinus infections.

Vibrio bacteria cause cellulitis and severe wound infections, which can spread to the bloodstream and lead to septic shock. They can invade the muscles and blood vessels and cause massive destruction of tissue. A man who contracted a *Vibrio* infection while clamming in Narragansett Bay a few years ago developed gangrene in his leg and had it amputated. A woman who had sexual intercourse in Galveston Bay developed *Vibrio* infection of the uterus.

Vibrio wound infections develop with lightning speed. They become red and swollen, and blood-containing, necrotizing blisters appear.

Treatment
Cleanse superficial coral cuts and other minor cuts and scrapes with antiseptic solution, apply a little antibiotic ointment, and cover with a light dressing. Large, ragged lacerations, deep puncture wounds, wounds with embedded foreign bodies, shark and

barracuda bites, and stingray wounds are at high risk for *Vibrio* infection. Cleanse them thoroughly with antiseptic solution, irrigate them with sterile saline, debride (remove) devitalized tissue, and administer prophylactic antibiotics. TMP-SMX, one double-strength tablet twice a day, or tetracycline, 500 mg every 6 hours, are good choices.

Established *Vibrio* wound infections can also be treated with TMP-SMX or tetracycline. Deep, necrotic infections are life- and limb-threatening, and require emergency surgical debridement. Arrange to have the patient evacuated to the nearest medical facility ASAP.

Prevention
Wear protective gloves when you handle fish and shellfish, and avoid contact with sea water when you have open wounds.

FRESHWATER BACTERIAL INFECTIONS

If you do most of your boating on inland lakes, you're likely to have an occasional encounter with *Aeromonas hydrophila*. This bug invades puncture wounds, cuts, and abrasions and causes cellulitis. Untreated or inadequately treated *Aeromonas* infections can, rarely, cause severe muscle and bone infections.

Treatment
Treatment consists of warm compresses, elevation of the infected part, and TMP-SMX, one double-strength tablet twice daily, or tetracycline, 250 mg every 6 hours.

Hot tub dermatitis is an infection with *Pseudomonas aeruginosa*, a bacterium that thrives in moist environments. You can catch it in a hot tub, whirlpool, or swimming pool. Hot water, chemical irritants, and well-hydrated skin set the stage for infection, which shows up a few hours to two days after exposure as a red, flat or bumpy, blistery rash on the trunk, limbs, and buttocks. The rash can be intensely itchy and may be associated with fever, malaise, and tender lymph nodes.

Treatment

Hot tub dermatitis resolves spontaneously in a week or two. You can control itching with calamine and diphenhydramine. Antibiotics are only necessary in severe cases.

SKIN PROBLEMS CAUSED BY DIVING EQUIPMENT

As if you scuba divers didn't have enough to worry about, what with recompression illness, middle-ear squeeze, sharks, and narcosis of the deep, your equipment can also make your life miserable.

"Mask burn," an allergic reaction to the material in your mask, can cause a dermatitis ranging in severity from a red facial imprint of the mask to a blistery, weeping rash. The mouthpiece of a regulator or snorkel can cause severe inflammation of the mouth and tongue. Some divers are allergic to their wet suits.

Treatment

Facial rashes respond well to cool Burow's solution compresses, 20 minutes four times a day, and 1% hydrocortisone ointment twice a day. Severe facial swelling and itching merit a course of prednisone (see "Sponge Dermatitis"). Quell the inflammation in your mouth and tongue with a 50:50 solution of milk of magnesia and diphenhydramine solution used as a mouthwash twice a day.

Prevention

If you know you are allergic to diving equipment, you'd be wise to invest in silicon rubber, hypoallergenic equipment.

SALTWATER SORES

Salt irritation of the skin, sun exposure, and chapping combine to cause painful salt sores. In a lifeboat or raft, the skin is repeatedly exposed to the sun and saltwater, and sores, ulcers, or boils are apt to develop in exposed areas. They can be prevented by keeping the skin dry, avoiding chafing, washing frequently with fresh water, and regular applications of mineral oil cream (Eucerin) containing 10% para-aminobenzoic acid (PABA) or fat or grease from dried fish or bird entrails.

．
．
．
．
．

8

DROWNING AND NEAR-DROWNING

A man who is not afraid of the sea will soon be drowned, he said, for he will be going out on a day when he shouldn't. But we do be afraid of the sea, and we do only be drownded now and again.

—John Millington Synge, *The Aran Islands*

The Aran Islands are three limestone slabs that thrust defiantly out of the Atlantic Ocean off the west coast of Ireland. For generations, the men of Aran took to the violent waters surrounding their islands in canoe-like *curraghs* to fish for cod, herring, ling, and basking sharks. Skilled and fearless boat handlers, Aranmen routinely maneuvered their craft through the 40- and 50-foot breakers that surge through Brannock Sound while returning from a day's fishing in the open Atlantic. The heavily laden boats were frequently swamped and their occupants drowned. Death at sea was such a common event that Aran fishermen wore wool "Aran sweaters" woven in distinctive family cable-stitch patterns so that their bodies could be identified when recovered.

Whether your boat is a curragh or a cutter, the only things separating you from a watery death are your boat-handling skills, your judgment, and the integrity of your craft. There are many routes to a watery death, including these.

1. *Falling overboard.* You can fall off a lurching boat in rough seas or be tossed over the side by a jibing boom or a giant wave. You can trip over gear strewn on the deck, lose your balance on a slick deck, or be yanked off the bow if your leg is caught in a bight in the anchor rode. And you can fall off your boat while relieving yourself over the transom (most male overboard victims are found with their flies open).

2. *Currents.* Whether attempting to swim ashore after falling overboard or swimming in the surf, you need to be wary of currents.

a. Rip currents. Strong onshore winds may temporarily dam water on the beach. When this water flows back out to sea along the path of least resistance (such as in a channel between two sandbars), a powerful rip current forms that flows a short distance out to sea. If you are caught in a rip current, *don't try to swim against it!* Remain calm and tread water until the rip current dissipates. Then swim parallel to the beach until you reach water that is moving shoreward. Rivers emptying into the sea behave very much like rip currents, as do the waters at the entrance to bays and inlets. If you remember not to fight these currents, you'll soon be out of them and heading for shore.

b. Along-shore currents. These currents flow parallel to the shore or at a slight angle away from the shore. If you are caught in an along-shore current, it may sweep you past a point of land and out to sea. The best strategy to escape an along-shore current is to swim with it, but at an angle toward the shore.

c. Undertow. Undertows are created when a wave runs back to sea under the succeeding wave. Although they are powerful, and can knock you off your feet, they are short-lived and won't suck you out to sea like some giant submarine vacuum cleaner. If you are knocked down by an undertow, allow it to roll you over the bottom for a few feet. Then head for the surface.

3. *Diving accidents.* See Chapter 14.

4. *Fish-human interactions.* You may be so severely injured after an encounter with a shark, barracuda, or man-of-war as to be unable to swim.

TERMINOLOGY

Before becoming immersed in a discussion of drowning and near-drowning, let's define a few terms. *Immersion* is the state of being in the water; *submersion* is the state of being under the water. *Drowning* is suffocation by submersion. *Near-drowning* is defined as survival for at least 24 hours after submersion. Drowning and near-drowning are *submersion incidents.*

RISK FACTORS

Submersion incidents are precipitated or aggravated by one or more of the following factors.

Head and Neck Injury

If you dive off your boat and strike your head on a rock, you're likely to sustain a head or neck injury. Loss of consciousness or a paralyzing neck injury will render you helpless, and you will die if you are not pulled out of the water immediately. Always probe the bottom for underwater obstructions before diving into unknown waters.

Alcohol

Alchemists in the Middle Ages thought that alcohol was the elixir of life. In fact, the word *whisky* comes from the Gaelic word *usquebaugh*, which means "water of life." Even today, many people believe that alcohol is a stimulant. It's not. It's a general anesthetic that depresses the central nervous system, jumbles and disorganizes thought, and impairs muscular coordination.

The mental functions most sensitive to alcohol are those that depend on training and previous experience. Alcohol also dulls discrimination, memory, concentration, and insight; raises the pain threshold; fragments sleep; and accelerates body cooling, increasing the risk of drowning secondary to immersion hypothermia (see below and Chapter 9). Little wonder that so many drownings are associated with drinking. (An Australian study revealed that two-thirds of men who drowned had been drinking beforehand.) Many Aran fishermen survived their battles with the Atlantic only to capsize their curraghs and drown while rowing home after stopping to have a few pints in the pub. (What do you do with a drunken sailor? You can "put him in the long boat and make him bale her," as the old sea chantey recommends, or you can follow the advice given in an early edition of the Royal Navy's *Ship's Captain's Medical Guide:*

Give the patient 30 grains of Sulphate of Zinc in a glass of beer, or any other liquid, to make him vomit. Get everything clear about his neck and waist, rest his head, well raised, on a wet swab and put him in the open air, properly protected from the cold.

Boating Accidents

Thirty percent of adult drownings occur after boating accidents. Injuries sustained in a crash with a pier or jetty may make it impossible for you to swim, or you may be thrown out of your boat during a capsize.

Hypothermia

Believe it or not, you won't die instantly if you fall into the cold waters of the North Atlantic, Lake Superior, or any other frigid body of water. But you will become *hypothermic* and drown if you aren't rescued within an hour or two. *Hypothermia* is the cooling of the body's core below 95 degrees, and you can become hypothermic in any water cooler than 77 degrees if you're immersed in it long enough. Hypothermia makes your muscles stiff and weak and impairs your coordination. The longer you are in cold water, the harder it will be for you to tread water or pull yourself out.

Underlying Medical Conditions

Epilepsy, heart disease, diabetes, chronic lung disease, and neurologic disorders all increase the risk of death by drowning. A seizure or heart attack will render you helpless in the water, and any chronic, debilitating disease will make it harder for you to stay afloat or pull yourself out of the water if you fall overboard.

THE MECHANISMS AND STAGES OF DROWNING

I have had two near-drowning experiences, and they were both terrifying. Theodate Pope, on the other hand, an American architect who was a passenger on the *Lusitania* when it was torpedoed by a U-boat on May 7, 1915, did not find her near-drowning experience as disturbing:

> *I . . . found a foothold on a roll of canvas used for deck shields and then jumped. . . . The next thing I realized was that I could not reach the surface, because I was being washed and whirled up against wood. I was swallowing and breathing the salt water, but felt no special discomfort nor anguish of mind—was strangely apathetic. . . . I closed my eyes and thought, "This is of course the end of life for me." . . . Then for perhaps half a minute I opened my eyes on a grey world. . . . I was surrounded and jostled by hundreds of frantic, screaming, shouting humans in this grey and watery inferno.*

> Theodate Pope, in a letter written to her mother shortly after she was rescued, reprinted in *American Heritage* in 1975

This is the sequence of events in drowning.

Stage I: Panic and Struggle

The victim panics and makes frantic efforts to get his head above water. If he can get his head out of the water, he hyperventilates. This stage lasts 20 to 60 seconds.

Stage II: Breath Holding

The victim closes his mouth and stops trying to breathe for about a minute.

Stage IIIA: Aspiration

The victim ceases to struggle; he swallows water and starts to vomit. He then aspirates the water and vomitus into his lungs, coughs violently, and gasps, drawing more water into the respiratory tree and lungs. This is known as "wet drowning."

Stage IIIB: Laryngospasm

About 10 to 15 percent of drowning victims don't aspirate water or vomitus. When water contacts the vocal cords, they go into a tight, prolonged spasm that blocks entry of water and vomitus into the lungs. This is called "dry drowning." Most survivors of submersion incidents are victims of dry drowning.

Stage IV: Respiratory Arrest

Anoxia (lack of oxygen) causes the victim to lose consciousness, and chest movement ceases.

Stage V: Death

The victim makes a few more ineffective efforts to breathe. Then the heart stops and he dies.

I can tell you from personal experience that it really happens this way. I fell into a well when I was four years old, and I'll never forget the sheer terror that gripped me as I thrashed and kicked wildly about, trying to breathe. I didn't see my life pass before my eyes, but I did see flashing lights of all kinds before I passed out. The next thing I remember was waking up in the farmhouse where my dad had carried me after pulling me out of the well just before I sank out of sight.

SUBMERSION PATHOPHYSIOLOGY— GETTING DOWN TO THE NITTY GRITTY

Unless you have gills, you can't breathe in oxygen and blow off carbon dioxide when you are underwater. Consequently, the concentration of oxygen in the blood and tissues plummets (hypoxemia), and carbon dioxide levels rise (hypercarbia). The brain cannot operate without a steady flow of oxygen; and hypercarbia causes narcosis, so you pass out after a few minutes. High levels of carbon dioxide lead to a surplus of acids in the blood and tissues (acidosis), which disrupts cellular metabolism in every organ. The damage done to the lungs by aspirated water depends on whether it is salt or fresh.

Freshwater Aspiration

Fresh water is hypotonic; it has a low concentration of dissolved salts relative to plasma, the liquid component of blood. When you aspirate fresh water, a portion of it is pulled into the plasma and into the red blood cells by osmosis. The blood thus becomes diluted, and the red blood cells may stretch until they pop.

Fresh water also destroys surfactant, the surface-tension-lowering substance that coats the inner surface of the lung and keeps the alveoli (small air chambers) open. As the alveoli collapse, hypoxemia worsens and the lungs become stiff and difficult to inflate.

Seawater Aspiration

Seawater contains a number of impurities and virulent bacteria and, ounce for ounce, is twice as lethal as fresh water. It's also more injurious to the lungs than fresh water. Seawater is three to four times more hypertonic than blood. Consequently, aspirated salt water draws plasma into the lungs through osmosis, and the alveoli become water-logged, a condition called "pulmonary edema"; it makes the lungs stiff and interferes with gas exchange in the lungs. Salt water also washes surfactant out of the alveoli, so the alveoli that don't fill with water collapse. As in freshwater aspiration, the end result of saltwater aspiration is hypoxemia, hypercapnia, and acidosis.

Brackish Water

Brackish water often contains chemical pollutants that can cause an intense inflammatory pneumonia. Sand, seaweed, mud, and sewage suspended in brackish water can be aspirated and can obstruct the airway.

Practically speaking, despite the different effects of fresh and salt water on the lungs, how *much* water is aspirated is more important than what *kind* of water. The end result is the same if the submersion victim isn't rescued and resuscitated: death by asphyxiation.

SPECIAL SITUATIONS

The Immersion Syndrome

Although rare, immersion in icy water can cause sudden death. In most cases, this results from the reflex gasp triggered by the shock of cold water on the skin. If you're under water when you gasp, you'll inhale a lungful of water and drown. Cold-induced reflex slowing of the heart leading to cardiac arrest also plays a role in many of these cases. But most people can survive for up to an hour in water less than 32 degrees Fahrenheit.

Cold-Water Drowning

Actually, your chances of surviving a submersion incident are greater in cold water. There have been many reports of children who survived and were successfully resuscitated after being submerged for as long as 66 minutes. Apparently these kids cooled so rapidly that they went into a "metabolic icebox" that slowed brain metabolism enough to prevent significant anoxic injury. Adults cool more slowly than children because of their lower surface-to-mass ratios and don't receive the full benefit of the metabolic icebox.

Shallow Water Blackout

Some people hyperventilate to saturate their tissues with oxygen before swimming under water. You can stay under longer using this technique, but it also may cause you to lose consciousness and drown. This is called "shallow-water blackout" or "breath-hold blackout" (see Chapter 14). Rapid breathing does increase the oxygen content of the blood, but it also lowers the carbon dioxide content. Carbon dioxide is the dominant breathing stimulus; its level will slowly build up again while you are swimming under water, but not as quickly as the oxygen content of the blood declines. When the oxygen level drops below a certain level, the lights go out and you drown.

RESCUING A DROWNING PERSON

What is the most dangerous creature in the sea? No, it's not the great white shark, the giant squid, or the killer whale. The most feared animal in any waters, fresh or salt, is the drowning human. He is an aggressive beast who will lunge at you and embrace you in a death hold that would defy the escape talents of the Great Houdini. Approach the drowning person very carefully, or you will both be in trouble. Theodate Pope had a close call with a drowning man shortly after she jumped off the sinking *Lusitania*:

> *A man insane with fright was clinging to my shoulders. I can see the panic in his eyes as he looked over my head. He had no life belt on and his weight was pulling me under again. Had I struggled against him, he probably would have clung to me. . . . I said "Oh, please don't" and then the water closed over me and I became unconscious again. He must have left me when he found me sinking under him.*

The safest way to approach the drowning person is the REACH, THROW, ROW, GO strategy.

1. REACH. First, extend a gaff, fishing pole, or oar to him. Let him grab the end and pull himself in. If you have a life ring or a rope, throw it to him and pull him in. (Just don't hit him on the head and knock him out!)

2. *THROW.* If he is beyond reach with a gaff or rope, throw him a life jacket, seat cushion, or any other object with enough flotation for him to keep his head out of water while you figure out how to get him to the boat or shore.

3. *ROW.* Next, you need to take your boat or a dinghy out to him and retrieve him from the water.

4. *GO.* If the victim is unconscious or too far away to reach with a pole or rope (and there is no boat available), and you are trained in water-rescue techniques, your only option is to swim out and get him. Use these techniques.

a. If the victim is cooperative, use the *tired swimmer's carry.* Approach him from the front, and instruct him to put his hands on your shoulders. Then use the breast stroke to return to shore.

b. If he is thrashing about wildly, swim to him underwater, turn him around so that he is facing away from you, and raise his head out of the water by lifting on his armpits. Then, place your hand under his jaw to keep his head out of the water, and allow his body to float to the surface and level off. Next, reach your arm around his chest (the cross-chest carry) and side-stroke to shore (see Figure 18). If he panics, clasp your hands and keep his face out of the water until he calms down. If he tries to crawl on top of you, let go of him and sink down into the water.

Treatment

Resuscitation techniques have come a long way in the past few decades. In Europe in the 1700s, the drowning victim was often placed face down on a trotting horse, or placed on or inside a barrel which was rolled back and forth in an effort to ventilate the lungs. The Society for Recovery of Drowned Persons was established in Amsterdam in 1767. Among the techniques they espoused to revive drowning victims were warming the victim by lighting a fire near him, burying him in warm sand, putting him in a warm bath, or putting him to bed with a couple of volunteers; removing aspirated water by tickling his throat with a feather to induce vomiting; stimulating him by rectal and oral fumigation

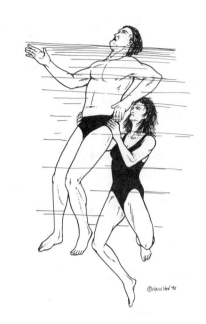

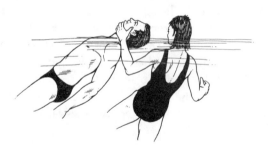

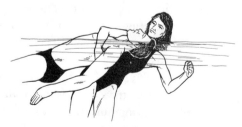

FIGURE 18
The cross-chest carry.

with tobacco smoke, or by squirting mixtures of oil, salt, and water into his mouth; and using a bellows to restore breathing or mouth-to-mouth breathing (which was not popular in those days of poor personal hygiene).

The modern approach to the submersion victim is as follows.

1. Remove him from the water as quickly as possible, taking care to splint his neck if there are grounds to suspect a neck injury, (e.g., a dive into shallow water, a surfing accident).

2. If the victim is not breathing, use the jaw-thrust technique (see Figure 1) to open his airway, clear any debris from his mouth and throat, and start mouth-to-mouth ventilation while still in the water. If he has no pulse, start chest compressions as soon as you can position him on a firm surface.

3. Most submersion victims aspirate very small amounts of water, so don't waste time doing drainage procedures.

4. Rewarm him if he is hypothermic.

5. Continue CPR (see Chapter 1) until you revive the victim or emergency medical personnel take over. If you're in a remote area, continue CPR until the victim has warmed to ambient temperature. Remember, the cold-water drowning victim is not dead until he's *warm* and dead. If the victim resumes breathing within 30 minutes of the start of rescue, he will very likely survive.

Prevention

1. Wear your personal flotation device at all times, and especially during rough weather. And keep that safety line hooked on the jackline.

2. Keep the lid on alcohol consumption, and bar illicit drugs from your vessel.

3. Install netting on your railings to keep children on board, or attach children to safety harnesses. And keep the decks clear of lines and gear that someone might trip over.

4. Inspect the bottom before you dive into unfamiliar waters. Don't rely on your depth recorder.

5. Operate your boat safely so as to avoid accidents.

6. Don't hyperventilate before swimming underwater.

7. Don't swim alone if you have a seizure disorder or any other serious medical problem.

8. If you become fatigued while swimming or treading water, use the drownproofing technique: Float face-down in the water with your chin on your chest, your waist slightly bent, and your arms out to the side. Use a short frog kick to raise your head high enough out of the water to take a quick breath. Then sink back into the water, relax, and repeat the cycle. This survival floating technique conserves energy, prevents aspiration of water, and may keep you alive until you are rescued or find something to cling to.

•
•
•
•
•

9

HYPOTHERMIA AND COLD-WATER IMMERSION

Her lips were red, her looks were free,
Her locks were yellow as gold:
Her skin was as white as leprosy,
The Night-mare LIFE-IN-DEATH was she,
Who thicks man's blood with cold.

—Samuel Taylor Coleridge, *The Rime of the Ancient Mariner*

On the morning of January 25, 1883, dory mates Howard Black-burn and Thomas Welch set out from the schooner *Grace L. Fears* to retrieve the trawls they had set earlier that day on the Burgeo Bank off the coast of Newfoundland. They had hauled in the last of their gear and were rowing back to the *Fears* when a winter storm swept in from the northwest. They lost sight of the ship in the blinding blizzard and spent that night at anchor. The snow stopped during the night, but cold arctic blasts and high seas continued to hammer them. They spent the next day hove to, bailing frantically to keep the dory afloat. Blackburn lost his mittens and a sock, and his hands froze to the oar handles. By night-fall, Welch was in a bad way and could no longer bail. He died during the night.

The storm abated on the morning of the third day, but the *Fears* was not on the horizon. Blackburn decided to row for shore, some 40 miles distant. He rowed all that day, and the friction of the oar handles wore away the frozen flesh on his hands. He put out a sea anchor that night and resumed rowing the next morning. He made landfall just before dusk and was taken in by a fisherman's family. Over the next five months, he slowly regained his health. However, he lost both heels and all his toes and fingers.

Hypothermia killed Thomas Welch. The cold turned Howard Blackburn's hands and feet into frozen stumps, but he was able to fight off hypothermia and exhaustion and survive his four-day ordeal in the North Atlantic. Why did Welch succumb to the cold and Blackburn survive?

HYPOTHERMIA—THE INVISIBLE KILLER

The cold found Thomas Welch in a dory in a North Atlantic blizzard. It was a cruel, penetrating cold that probed with icy claws and searched like a hunger-crazed wolf for the warmth that sustained his body and spirit. It sucked the warmth from his marrow and left him stiff and lifeless in the bottom of the dory.

The cold will find you, too, someday, so you'd better "know your enemy." Hypothermia is a drop in body temperature to below 95 degrees Fahrenheit. The body's thermostat is set at around 98.6 degrees, the optimal temperature for all the body's life-sustaining chemical reactions. When the core temperature varies more than a few degrees up or down, cellular metabolism becomes unhinged and the organ systems start to malfunction. To stay at around 98.6 degrees, the body must balance heat production and heat losses.

Routes of Heat Loss

1. *Radiation* is the transfer of heat from the body to cooler objects by electromagnetic waves. Normally, radiation accounts for 50 to 70 percent of body heat loss.

2. *Conduction* is the direct transfer of heat from the body to a cooler medium. Conductive heat losses are minimal in air but are substantial during cold-water immersion. Because water has a specific heat four thousand times greater than air, and thermal conductivity twenty-five times greater, your body will cool more than a hundred times faster in water than in air of the same temperature.

3. *Convection* is heat loss secondary to the disruption of the thin layer of warm air or water next to the skin. As the body gives off heat, it warms a small strip of air or water next to the skin.

When exposed to wind or moving water, this thin strip is disturbed, and a new strip is heated at the expense of body heat loss. This is the basis of the wind-chill factor, the increased cooling of skin when exposed to wind. (The amount of heat loss varies with the square of the wind velocity.)

4. *Evaporation* of water from the skin and lungs accounts for 30 percent of body heat loss in the cold and a much higher percentage when the skin is wet and exposed to high winds.

Heat Generation and Preservation

Your body would stay at ambient (surrounding) temperature if it didn't have the means to generate and conserve heat. When the surface of the body starts to cool, chilled blood and signals from thermoreceptors in the skin alert the thermoregulatory center in an area of the brain called the "hypothalamus." The hypothalamus activates the sympathetic nervous system, which mediates these *involuntary* defensive reactions to the cold.

1. *Constriction* of blood vessels in the skin and muscles, and *dilation* of the vessels in the brain and internal organs. This creates a cool outer shell that insulates a warm internal core.

2. *Shivering,* which increases heat production up to 500 percent. Shivering starts when the core temperature drops below 98.6 degrees and stops when it reaches about 86 degrees or the muscles run out of fuel.

3. Inhibition of *sweating,* limiting evaporative heat losses.

4. Increased *blood pressure, heart rate,* and *respiratory rate.*

5. A 25 percent increase in the *basal metabolic rate* by an increase in muscle tone throughout the body.

Your *brain* is your most powerful weapon in the fight against hypothermia. *Voluntary* defenses against the cold include:

1. *Exercise.* You can generate twice as much heat per hour exercising as you can by shivering, up to 1000 kcal an hour if you are well-conditioned. Howard Blackburn survived his four-day ordeal in the North Atlantic because he stayed busy rowing and bailing his dory. Thomas Welch might have survived if he had helped with the rowing.

2. *Clothing.* We humans don't have thick coats of fur or water-repellant feathers to protect us against the elements, but we *are* able to don protective clothing. Air is one of the best insulators, and layers of clothing that create thin air pockets provide the best protection against the cold.

3. *Seeking Shelter.* Going down into the cabin, for example, will conserve body heat.

Causes and Predisposing Factors

1. *Exposure.* You don't have to be sailing in an ice field to become hypothermic. Cool temperatures, low humidity, high winds, and inadequate or wet clothing can all lead to hypothermia in any season and at any latitude. (I became hypothermic while sailing on Lake Michigan one cool, breezy summer evening some years ago. I was clad only in a swimsuit, and after a couple of hours, I became lethargic and my muscles became stiff and sluggish. I don't know how I made it back to shore.)

2. *Age.* Because of their high surface-area-to-mass ratio, children lose a lot of body heat through radiation. Infants have poorly developed shivering mechanisms and little fat to insulate them. Elderly people are predisposed to hypothermia because they have less fat and muscle to insulate them from the cold and their cardiovascular systems don't respond as well to cold stress.

3. *Immersion.* Cold water pulls heat from the body like a magnet.

4. *Trauma and immobility.* If you break your leg when a curling breaker crashes over the stern and slams you down the companionway, you're not going to generate much heat through exercise for a while, and you'll have a tough time getting out of your wet clothes.

5. *Drugs and alcohol.* Alcohol is a general anesthetic. It may blind you to the fact that you are becoming hypothermic and prevent you from donning warm clothes or seeking shelter. And it dilates the vessels in the skin, giving you that warm glow after a couple of drinks. But that glow comes at the expense of heat loss, as warm blood from the core perfuses the cold shell. Alcohol may inhibit shivering, and alcohol and other drugs impair your judgment and coordination, which opens the door to mistakes and injury.

The Signs and Symptoms of Hypothermia

Mild Hypothermia
(90 to 95 Degrees Fahrenheit)

The victim is usually shivering, and his skin is cool to the touch. His speech is slurred, he moves slowly, and he complains of feeling weak and fatigued. He may be confused and apathetic, and have difficulty handling sheets and lines, or holding binoculars or navigational instruments.

Severe Hypothermia
(Below 90 Degrees Fahrenheit)

The victim's skin is cold to the touch, blue, and mottled. He may become dejected and lose the will to live. As the core temperature drops below 90 degrees, he becomes progressively more confused and lethargic, until he lapses into a coma. He stops shivering, and he may hallucinate and act inappropriately, taking off his clothes or jumping off an overturned boat. His pulse and respiration slow, and lethal heart rhythms may develop. He becomes profoundly weak and tired, his muscles become rigid, and he stops moving.

Detecting Hypothermia

Hypothermia is not as easy to diagnose as seasickness. It has an insidious onset, and you have to be on the lookout for it when the wind is Force 5 and the seas are breaking over your bow, throwing blankets of cold water across the cockpit, soaking you and your crew to the skin. *Shivering* is the most obvious sign of hypothermia, but you should also suspect it in anyone who has been exposed to the cold, wind, and spray and is sluggish or

confused, or has difficulty handling lines. You can take the victim's temperature, but most clinical thermometers don't register
below 96 degrees.

IMMERSION HYPOTHERMIA

As the *Titanic* slid into the black depths of the North Atlantic
that fateful April night in 1912, hundreds of men leaped into the
freezing water in a desperate attempt to save themselves. Most of
them wore life jackets, but only the few who were picked up by
lifeboats survived. The rest died in the water before the *Carpathia*
arrived on the scene two hours after the sinking.

The water was warmer than the air that night, yet none of the
people in the boats died. That may seem odd, unless you're familiar with the concept of *cold water immersion*.

Falling into freezing water is *not* synonymous with instant death.
Any member of the Polar Bear club can tell you that. But if you
remain in the water more than an hour or so, you'll develop
hypothermia, lose consciousness, and drown.

Into the Drink—What Happens

If you go over the rail into the cold waters of Lake Champlain,
the Drake Passage, or the Skagerrak, your first reaction will be
a huge, involuntary gasp, and then you'll hyperventilate for a
minute or so. If you are underwater when you gasp, you may
aspirate a large amount of water into your lungs and asphyxiate.
(You can short circuit the gasp reflex by entering the water slowly
if you are abandoning a sinking vessel.) If you have a weak heart,
the shock of the cold water may cause your heart to go into a
lethal arrhythmia. Sudden death on entry into cold water is called
the *immersion syndrome*. It's quite rare.

Hyperventilation causes carbon dioxide to accumulate in the
blood, which in turn constricts the cerebral blood vessels. Inadequate blood flow to the brain may lead to confusion, loss of coordination, fainting, and drowning. And the excessive respiratory

stimulation lowers your breath-holding ability from a normal average of 60 seconds to only 15 to 25 seconds in 15-degree water. Not good if you're trapped under a capsized boat.

Just as in hypothermia in general, during cold-water immersion the circulation to the skin and muscles shuts down while blood flow to the brain and vital organs in the chest and abdomen increases. This is a mixed blessing in cold water because the muscles become stiff and weak. Anyone immersed in icy water for more than 5 minutes will have difficulty swimming, donning a personal flotation device (PFD), climbing a ladder, or hanging onto a line. He'll lose fine-motor control and may be unable to operate signaling devices or inflate a PFD or life raft.

After 15 to 20 minutes in freezing water, the core starts to cool as heat is conducted to the cold shell. The victim becomes confused and lethargic. He may jump off an overturned boat, attempt to swim to a distant shore, or take off his PFD. Intense cold may destroy his will to live. On the plus side, as the core temperature drops, the brain's metabolism slows, and it becomes more tolerant of hypoxia (deficient oxygen). Some people have been successfully resuscitated after being submerged for more than 40 minutes in cold water.

The Great Escape—Heat Loss in Cold Water

The big difference between hypothermia in air and immersion hypothermia is that cold water sucks the heat out of your body like a vacuum cleaner. You may take all day to become hypothermic topside on a 40-degree day, but only an hour and a half in 40-degree water.

Different parts of the body cool at different rates. The digits and limbs cool most rapidly because of their high surface-to-volume ratio. The head dissipates heat readily because of its high blood flow and poor insulation. The front and sides of the chest are poorly insulated and cool rapidly, and the groin and neck are heat sieves, because large blood vessels lie just under the skin.

Here are the factors that determine your cooling rate in water, in order of importance.

1. *Water temperature.* The colder the water, the faster you will cool.

2. *Body fat.* Have you ever wondered why whales and seals don't become hypothermic? Their bodies are insulated by thick layers of blubber (fat), which have a very poor blood supply and is an excellent insulator. Researchers have shown that doubling the skin-fold thickness halves the cooling rate. This is one situation where you can feel good about being fat. That blubber may save your life.

3. *Clothing.* Insulated clothing designed to trap small pockets of air near the skin is of no value in water. Water quickly saturates the clothing and obliterates the air pockets. And small layers of warm water are flushed away as soon as they form. However, multiple layers of heavy clothing can increase survival time in cold water by 30 to 40 percent. *Wet garments* (wet suits, insulated coveralls, and thermal flotation jackets) limit the flow of water between skin and clothing and can greatly increase survival time. Float coats reduce cooling by 40 to 50 percent and double survival time. *Dry garments* (survival suits) employ impermeable neck, wrist, and ankle seals and a water-tight zipper to keep water out. Snug-fitting vest-type PFDs provide some protection.

4. *Sea state.* It can be tough to keep your mouth out of the water in rough seas. And wind and spray accelerate cooling.

5. *Behavior.* When you swim or tread water, two undesirable things happen: warm blood from the core flows into the muscles and you lose your shell insulation, and water moving over your body increases convective heat losses. You will cool up to 50 percent faster if you exercise in the water. Most people can't swim more than a half mile in 50-degree water, so trying to swim for shore is rarely a wise move. Your best bet is to get as much of your body out of the water as possible. Climb up on the hull of your boat if it is still afloat. Evaporative heat loss may make you feel colder out of the water, but you will cool much more slowly than you would in the water. If you can't get out of the water, limit skin exposure to the water by assuming the HELP (Heat-Escape-Lessening Posture) position (see Figure 19). If you are with a group of people, huddle together and maximize upper body contact.

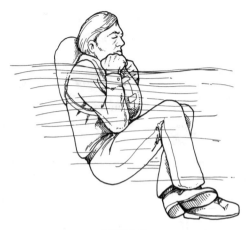

FIGURE 19
The HELP (*Heat-Escape-Lessening Posture*) position.

6. *Body type.* Children and tall, thin persons cool relatively quickly because of their high surface-to-volume ratio. Big people cool more slowly than little people.

7. *Shivering.* Shivering helps to retard core cooling, but it generally stops at 86 degrees.

8. *Gender.* Women have a higher percentage of body fat than men, but they are smaller. The net result is equivalent cooling rates for men and women.

9. *Fitness.* Fit people are stronger and have more stamina. But they also have less fat, so the survival value of fitness is moot.

10. *Alcohol.* Alcohol may be the reason you enter the water in the first place. If you're three sheets to the wind, you'll probably drown. Moderate amounts of alcohol don't affect the cooling rate in cold water.

COLD-WATER SURVIVAL

Survival Time

The good news about cold-water immersion is that you will survive longer than you think. That's also the bad news. Floating in a fetal position in ice water is not one of life's great pleasures. But as cold as you might feel on the outside, your core won't start to cool for at least 15 or 20 minutes, even in ice water. But once it does, your core temperature will plummet like a sinking ore carrier until, after an hour and 15 minutes, it reaches 86 degrees. At that point, you will very likely lose consciousness and drown, or die of an irregular heartbeat. The average, thinly dressed person can survive for 2.5 hours in 50-degree water, and for up to 12 hours in 68-degree water.

Cold-Water Survival Techniques

Charles Joughin, chief baker on the *Titanic*, had an intuitive understanding of how to survive cold water immersion:

> The deck was now listing too steeply to stand on, and Joughin slipped over the starboard rail and stood on the actual side of the ship. He worked his way up the side . . . until he reached the white-painted steel plates of the poop deck. He now stood on the rounded stern end of the ship, which had swung high in the air some 150 feet above the water. . . . [He] casually tightened his lifebelt . . . [and] was beginning to puzzle over his position when he felt the stern beginning to drop under his feet—it was like taking an elevator. As the sea closed over the stern, Joughin stepped off into the water. He didn't even get his head wet. He paddled off into the night, little bothered by the freezing water. For over an hour he bobbed about, moving his arms and legs just enough to keep upright. . . . [Then] they pulled him in [to a lifeboat].
>
> —Walter Lord, *A Night to Remember*

Joughin did all the right things. He didn't enter the water until the last possible moment, he kept his head out of the water, and he moved as little as possible. True, he didn't assume the HELP position, but it hadn't been invented yet in 1912. And we don't know how he was attired when he stepped with such great timing off the stern of the sinking *Titanic*. They didn't have survival suits in those days, but Joughin could have improved his chances of surviving a moonlight swim in the frigid North Atlantic by donning every stitch of heavy clothing he owned, including a waterproof outer garment.

Joughin never had the option, but you may consider swimming to shore if it's within a reasonable distance (less than half a mile), you are an excellent swimmer, and you are wearing a PFD. If you don't know how to swim, the drown-proofing technique (see Chapter 8) may save your life. However, this requires you to immerse your head in the water and to actively move your limbs and trunk. You will cool 80 percent quicker using the drown-proofing technique than you would if you were simply floating in a PFD. But if the alternative is drowning, go for it.

Psychology can be as important as physiology when you are fighting for your life in the cold. Thomas Welch's last words to his dory mate Howard Blackburn were: "Howard, what is the use, we cannot last until morning. We might as well go first as last." He died of hypothermia a few hours later. Charles Joughin, on the other hand, had a positive attitude as he entered the water, and he survived. A powerful will to live is of supreme importance in cold-water immersion.

RESCUE AND FIRST AID

The person who goes over the side and is retrieved quickly, and is alert, shivering, and able to assist in his rescue, will be only mildly hypothermic. Have him go down into the cabin, put on dry clothing, wrap himself in a blanket, and sip on a hot drink. He'll be back in action in an hour or so.

Some years ago, sixteen Danish fishermen jumped into the icy waters of the North Sea when their trawler sank in a storm. They were in the water for a couple of hours before being rescued. They walked across the deck of the rescue vessel and went down into the galley to warm up. Every one of them died of hypothermia.

If your man has been in the drink for more than 20 to 30 minutes, is lightly dressed, and has been swimming or treading water, assume that he is *profoundly* hypothermic. Especially if he's blue, stuporous, and not shivering. Approach him as though he were a contact mine. His heart is cold and irritable, and if you handle him roughly you can precipitate ventricular fibrillation. And if you allow him to move under his own power, or try to rewarm him, he may suffer from "afterdrop" (a sudden drop in core temperature when cold, venous blood surges back to the heart from cold muscles). Have a man get in the water to assist him and, if possible, use a sling and hoist to bring him back on board.

Hypothermia causes hypotension (low blood pressure), but this is balanced somewhat by the hydrostatic squeeze on the parts of the victim's body that are immersed. His blood pressure may plummet like a sounding line if he is suddenly removed from the water, and he may collapse and die. Keep him as horizontal as possible while hoisting him from the water, and place him in a supine position once you get him on board.

Treatment

1. Check the ABCs. Check his respiration and pulse, and make sure he has a good airway. (See Chapter 1.) If he is pulseless and not breathing, start CPR, and continue until you are exhausted or are relieved by rescue personnel. Hypothermia victims have been successfully resuscitated after 3 hours of CPR. Do *not* perform CPR if he has any pulse and respiration, no matter how feeble. If he is found floating face down, treat him as a near-drowning (see Chapter 8).

2. *Examine* him from head to toe. His pupils may be fixed and dilated, but hypothermia victims aren't dead until they are "warm and dead."

3. *Prevent further heat loss.* Take him into the cabin, remove his wet clothing, gently dry his skin, and cover him with blankets or a sleeping bag.

4. *Apply hot packs* to his neck, armpits, trunk, and groin, or have two people get undressed from the waist up, get into bed with him, and maintain close chest-to-chest contact. Be careful not to burn his skin, and do *not* apply heat to any other areas.

5. *Administer warmed (104-degree) intravenous fluids* if possible.

6. *Don't* give him alcohol or any other drink. Hot drinks won't warm him, and he might aspirate if he is not fully alert.

7. Have someone *call the Coast Guard* while you are attending to the victim.

•
•
•
•
•

10

MAN OVERBOARD

Obscurest night involved the sky,
The Atlantic billows roared,
When such a destined wretch as I,
Washed headlong from onboard
Of friends, of hope, of all bereft,
His floating home for ever left.

—William Cowper, *The Castaway*

On Friday, September 29, 1989, I attended the annual scientific meeting of the Wilderness Medical Society in Stratton, Vermont. One of the speakers was Dr. Ray Brown, a surgeon and veteran sailor from Annapolis, Maryland, who lectured on the problem of man overboard. In his talk, he said that recovery of a man overboard in storm conditions was almost impossible; in moderate weather conditions it *might* be possible with training and practice in man overboard procedures. In light of these facts, Dr. Brown concluded that ". . . the best medical management is anticipation and prevention of man overboard by wearing a safety harness. *Stay on the boat!*"

On Sunday, October 1, two days later, I came across the following item in *The Burlington Free Press:*

> BLOCK ISLAND, R. I.—*Coast Guard officials suspended*
> *their search Saturday for a 65-year-old Maryland man who*
> *apparently fell overboard while sailing.*
>   *Seaman Robert Baccarie said Raymond N. Brown, a*
> *doctor from Annapolis, Md., apparently fell off a boat he*
> *was on with his wife and four other people. . . .*

Dr. Brown had just taken delivery of a new Alden 50 in Portsmouth, Rhode Island, and was sailing home to Annapolis. He came off the midnight-to-4 A.M. watch as they were entering The

Race, a stretch of strong currents and turbulent water between the eastern tip of Long Island and Block Island. Dr. Brown went below, slipped off his harness, and consulted his charts. He returned to the cockpit, made a course correction, and then went forward to inspect the jib, which was fluttering. Suddenly, a wave caused the boat to lurch. The main boom jibed and knocked Dr. Brown over the side. He was never seen again, despite an exhaustive search by his crew and the Coast Guard.

As a surgeon and a sailor, Ray Brown had to know that disaster strikes when you least expect it. And surely he realized that compulsive attention to detail and the refusal to cut corners are keys to success both in the operating room and in offshore sailing. But Ray Brown let his guard down for a moment, and he paid the ultimate price for his momentary indiscretion.

The leading cause of accidental boating fatalities is people falling off their boats. The proximate cause of most of these man-overboard accidents is a sudden lurch of the boat, an unexpected large wave, or a misstep. These are all problems that can be anticipated and avoided through strict adherence to safety rules, deployment of modern man-overboard equipment, and by regular practice of man-overboard procedures.

Prevention

1. *Keep the deck and cockpit uncluttered.* Your deck and cockpit area shouldn't be an obstacle course. Coil all sheets and lines, and secure spinnaker poles, life rafts, and other gear to the deck or cabin top.

2. *Don't urinate over the side at night or when the sea is rough.* Most men who fall overboard are found with their flies open. When the waves are short and steep, a sailboat becomes a seesaw, with great vertical excursions of the bow and stern, and little up-and-down motion at the beam. Many men have gone into the drink trying to relieve themselves off a heaving stern while hanging onto the backstay with one hand. Don't get caught with your fly down!

3. *Use personal flotation devices (PFDs).* You should be a Captain Bligh when it comes to PFDs. Insist that everyone who boards your boat immediately slip one on, old salts as well as landlubber guests. A PFD not only helps the man overboard keep his head out of the water, it also provides some protection against hypothermia, which is a threat to anyone who falls overboard in most American inland and coastal waters.

PFDs come in various types to suit different needs. The offshore sailor should wear an *offshore life jacket*. Although bulky, they are quite buoyant and will hold an unconscious person's face out of the water. The *nearshore buoyancy vest* is an awkward device that may or may not turn the wearer's face up in the water. The *flotation aid* is a vest or float coat that, while not designed to turn the wearer's face up in the water, is quite comfortable. The *throwable device* is a flotation cushion, life ring, or horseshoe ring that should be kept in the cockpit to throw to a man overboard. *Hybrid devices* are Mae Wests—carbon dioxide-inflated life preservers combined with a safety harness or float coat.

All PFDs should have an attached plastic whistle. Whistles are louder and more directional than screams, and less tiring for someone who is fighting the waves, cold, and exhaustion. PFDs should also have a strobe or waterproof light attached for nighttime and a signal mirror for daytime use.

4. *Use safety harnesses and jacklines.* There should be one safety harness for each crew member, and he should always wear it at night and when a high sea is running. The harness should fit snugly and have a stainless steel clip at either end of a 6-foot lifeline. The bitter end of the lifeline attaches to a jackline running at deck level from the cockpit to the bow, and the other end attaches to the harness at shoulder height.

Harnesses, like seat belts or air bags in a car, are not foolproof. The harness may pull off, the wearer may be unable to unclip himself before a sinking boat pulls him under, or the victim may be dragged underwater and drowned by the forward motion of the boat. Solo circumnavigator Dodge Morgan discovered the fallibility of lifelines when he fell off his sloop *American Promise* while crossing the southern Indian Ocean:

> My arm and face dip in and out of the freezing water as I
> chip and scrape. Then the boat takes a lurch, my boots slip

on the ladder rung, and my feet fly. Suddenly, I am looking up at PROMISE's stern—it is five feet away and departing, a stupefying sight. The forty degree water seems to take a long time to soak through my foul weather gear and pile pants and jacket and long underwear to my skin. When it does, I can't breathe. I am eight feet behind PROMISE when I begin to follow along obediently in her wake. My personal lifeline is clipped to the boarding ladder and it straightens out and holds. Then, almost as if PROMISE understands my predicament, her sails luff and she stands straight up in front of me. Then I can haul myself back to her and climb the boarding ladder. . . . I remember being told how even a strong man cannot pull himself upstream on his lifeline through a six knot wake fully dressed.

—Dodge Morgan, *The Voyage of American Promise*

5. *Wear shoes.* Deck shoes with corrugated rubber soles give you traction on wet or dry decks. Rubber-soled socks were designed for wind-surfers, but they grip the deck like Velcro. They may look silly, but they work.

MAN-OVERBOARD EQUIPMENT

The Overboard Pole

An *overboard pole* is a 6- to 8-foot-long pole that is mounted on the backstay and is jettisoned either immediately after the man overboard alarm is raised, or after the first attempt to recover the victim, if that attempt fails. The pole should have a flag at the top, a built-in strobe, a radar reflector, and a sea anchor so that the pole drifts at the same speed as the man overboard. You should attach an inflatable PFD to the pole, as well as a waterproof bag containing four red minirockets.

The Man Overboard Module

The *Man Overboard Module* is an overboard pole plus a survival platform. It can be deployed quickly by either a lanyard or an electric release mechanism positioned near the helmsman, and provides buoyancy as well as visibility to the person in the water.

MAN OVERBOARD! THE FIRST THIRTY SECONDS

The "Man overboard" alarm should trigger an explosion of activity on any vessel at sea. A crew member has gone over the side and will be swallowed by the sea if his shipmates don't respond reflexively with a coordinated and well-rehearsed series of activities designed to reunite vessel and victim in the shortest possible time. Successful recovery of a man overboard requires planning, teamwork, excellent boat handling skills, and, at times, great courage, as demonstrated by the crew of the *Grace Harwar*, a Finnish square-rigger, when she rounded Cape Horn in 1929:

> The next day one of the boys was swept overboard by a big sea. . . . We jammed the wheel hard down and brought her up, moaning and shivering. . . . One of us had gone aloft to the mizzen top to see where the lad had gone—if he was still afloat. We saw he had grasped a life buoy flung to him, and he still lived. Night was coming on, with rain squalls and a gale in the offing. But we got the boat over, and six volunteers leaped into it. . . . No one hung back.
>
> We dropped astern. The boat seemed a futile thing, rising and falling in the big seas. From troughs we saw the ship's royal yards sweep wild arcs through the gray sky, then not even that. We had no idea where the boy was. Maybe it was madness to look.
>
> We pulled this way and that, hopelessly; yet we could not go back. It began to rain heavily. None of us had oilskins. Frenchman was in his underwear, just as he had come from his bunk. . . . Sjoberg . . . had been laid up with neuralgia. But now he pulled at his oar, coatless and wet through. We did not want to lose another shipmate to Cape Horn.
>
> The mate . . . swept the sea with his eyes. There was a chance we would not find the ship again if the squall came down heavily and shut her out. That had happened with the

*Swedish bark Staut. She had put out a boat to save a boy,
a squall came down, and she lost everybody—the boy
overboard, those who went to rescue him, the boat. We
remembered that.*

*Then in the last moment of light we saw him. He was on
a crest only three seas away! We had been on the point of
giving up. Now we lay to heartily and pulled him in over the
stern and went back to the ship, which had watched us and
was running slowly downwind toward us. The boy was
unconscious and nearly frozen to death, but he lived.*

—Captain Alan Villiers, *Men, Ships and the Sea*

You'll probably never be called upon to rescue a man overboard in such dreadful conditions. But even under the best of circumstances, with calm winds, smooth seas, and the latest in lifesaving technology, recovery of a man in the drink will test your nerve and seamanship. Time is of the essence; what you do in the first half minute will determine success or failure. Here is the procedure to follow when a man goes over the side.

1. *Yell out "Man overboard"* at the top of your lungs three times.

2. *Start to count off the seconds.* A sailboat moving at 6 knots travels about 10 feet per second. By counting off the seconds, you can keep track of the distance separating the man in the water and the boat.

3. *Heave flotation cushions over the side.* Even if the victim can't reach them, they will mark the approximate site of his entry into the water. (Some authorities recommend immediate jettisoning of the overboard pole, but by the time you get it in the water, the boat will have travelled several hundred feet farther from the victim. Better to hold off on deploying the pole until after the first pass, if it is unsuccessful.)

4. *Note the boat's heading* before turning.

5. Assign a crew member to *point at the man in the water* and continue to count off the seconds. He should know the boat's course, and never take his eyes off the victim.

6. Make a *crash stop.* Come about and get the boat headed downwind as quickly as possible. There are two ways of doing this.

a. Quick-Stop maneuver. After sounding the man overboard alarm and throwing cushions into the water, turn the bow into and through the wind and let the headsails back. Lower the headsail and sail downwind until the man overboard is aft of the beam. Then jibe and approach him from leeward at an angle of 45 to 60 degrees off the wind. Throw him a heaving line and pull him to the boat.

b. Jibe maneuver. This is similar to the quick-stop maneuver. The only difference is that you stop the boat by heading the bow *off* the wind. Then jibe the mainsail, head right up into the wind, and coast to windward while lowering the jib. If the turn is executed properly, you will come to a stop just to the leeward of the man in the water. (The quick-stop maneuver is the technique of choice. The jibe maneuver is dangerous, takes more time to execute, and can be difficult to execute; it should be reserved for situations where you are sailing without a headsail, or for boats that don't turn well in light or strong breezes.)

Use the engine if you want, but be careful that lines and sheets hanging over the side don't foul the prop. And when you bring the victim alongside, make sure he knows that the engine is running.

SECTOR SEARCH

If you don't sight the man overboard on your first pass, jettison the overboard pole (if you haven't already done so) and start a systematic, six-sector search for the swimmer. In doing this, you will describe a pattern of three equilateral triangles having contingent corners at the pole. Proceed as follows.

1. Start at the overboard pole and move in a straight line away from it for twice the time elapsed between the accident and the deployment of the pole (alternatively, travel 0.5 nautical miles or 5 minutes).

2. Then turn 120 degrees to starboard, and run the same time or distance. Make another 120-degree turn, and run through the center of the circle and past it the same time or distance. After your fourth pass by the pole, turn left 120 degrees and continue this routine until you have completed the search pattern.

3. Make speed and distance adjustments for the wind. The pole is probably moving through the water faster than the victim, so make your first run straight up into the wind.

4. Broadcast "Mayday" on VHF Channel 16.

5. Have one crewman scan the sea within 1,000 feet of your boat, and another with binoculars search beyond 1,000 feet.

6. Stop, look, and listen if you come across the cushions that you heaved over the side right after the man-overboard alarm. Sound your horn and listen some more.

RECOVERY

Finding a man who has fallen overboard can be like finding a needle in a haystack; getting him back on board can be as tricky as putting a ship in a bottle. If the sea is calm, and he is in good condition, you can pull him to the boat with a heaving line and he can use a swimming ladder to climb aboard, or you can haul him on board. If he is weak or unconscious, the seas are rough, or the sides of the vessel too high, you'll have to slip a sling under his arms, hook it to a halyard, and hoist him aboard. You can rig up a sling by tying a large bowline in the end of a line, and a smaller one that you can attach to the main halyard. Then hoist him onto the deck with the halyard winch.

The Seattle sling (Lifesling) is a combination heaving line and hoisting sling. It's a horseshoe-shaped float attached to a length of floating polypropylene line. Use it as follows.

• Approach the swimmer at an angle of 45 to 60 degrees off the wind, jettison the sling, and trail it behind the boat.

• Sail to a position just downwind of the victim, and make a wide turn into the wind when he is astern of you.

• Tack, head off the wind again, and circle around the swimmer. He should grab and hang onto the Lifesling at this point.

• Stop the boat, head to the wind, and drop the mainsail.

• Haul the victim to the boat and hoist him aboard. (If he has been in the drink for 15 minutes or more, assume that he is hypothermic. Someone may need to get into the water to help him, because he may be confused, weak, and unable to coordinate his limb movements. Handle the potentially hypothermic swimmer gently—rough treatment can cause cardiac arrest!)

11
SURVIVAL AT SEA

*They that go down to the sea in ships, that do business in
  great waters;*
*These see the works of the Lord, and his wonders in the
  deep.*
*For he commandeth, and raiseth the stormy wind, which
  lifteth up the waves thereof.*
*They mount up to the heaven, they go down again to the
  depths: their soul is melted because of trouble.*
*They reel to and fro, and stagger like a drunken man, and
  are at their wit's end.*
*Then they cry unto the Lord in their trouble, and he bringeth
  them out of their distresses.*
*He maketh the storm a calm, so that the waves thereof are
  still.*
*Then are they glad because they be quiet; so he bringeth them
  unto their desired haven.*

Holy Bible, Psalm 107, Verses 23–30

Jumping off a sinking vessel in mid-ocean and entrusting your fate
to a rubber raft can only be compared to one other wrenching
human experience: birth. One moment you are safe and secure in
a warm, familiar environment; the next you are thrust violently
into a cold, tempestuous, and hostile world. But, unlike the new-
born, who is helpless, as a castaway, you hold your fate largely in
your own hands. With a seaworthy raft, a reasonable supply of
food and water, a few threads of clothing, and a little luck, you
may live for a few days. But to survive a prolonged ordeal in the
harshest, most punishing milieu on earth, you'll need more than a
survival bag. You'll need the courage and resourcefulness of Ulysses, the tenacity of Captain Ahab, and an unconquerable will to
live. Without these inner resources, you will wither and die under
the combined assault of sun, sea, thirst, and starvation.

PREPAREDNESS

The immediate objective in abandoning ship is to avoid drowning. Once you get into your survival craft, thirst, hunger, exposure, and depression become your mortal enemies. These relentless foes can ravage your body and corrode your soul. Douglas MacArthur once said, "Preparation is the key to victory." It's also the key to survival at sea.

Personal Preparation

The most important factor in surviving shipwreck is the ability to swim well. If you aren't a strong swimmer, you should at least develop some proficiency in treading water and drownproofing (see Chapter 8).

Knowledge is power. Learn all you can about first aid, small-boat handling, navigation, and food and water procurement before heading for blue water. You can glean a great deal of practical advice on survival at sea from reading Steven Callahan's *Adrift* and Dougal Robertson's *Survive the Savage Sea.*

Develop a Plan

Regularly rehearse abandon-ship procedures, and assign the following tasks to specific crew members.

- Transferring food and water supplies into the survival craft.
- Transferring the survival bag into the survival craft.
- Taking a navigational fix and recording it.
- Sending distress signals.
- Launching the survival craft.

Equipment

Your life raft should come equipped with stores of food and water, an EPIRB (Emergency Position-Indicating Radio Beacon), space blankets, a drogue, a solar still, polypropylene line, paddles, flares, a raft-repair kit, a medical kit, fishing tackle, and a flashlight. That's a good start, but not enough stuff for a prolonged ordeal. Supplement it with a survival bag containing these items.

• Food: dates, raisins, figs, granola bars, beef jerky, beef extracts, crackers and peanut butter, and canned fruit, meats, and vegetables.

• Another solar still or a reverse osmosis desalinator.

• A juice press to squeeze fluid out of bird and fish flesh.

• Two sponges.

• A radar reflector.

• A collapsible rubber basin and a plastic drinking cup.

• Polypropylene heaving line (¼ inch), 100 feet.

• Clothing: long-sleeved shirts, pants, hats with brims; survival suits and winter clothing when appropriate.

• Sunglasses, sunscreen, and sunblock.

• A medical kit (see Chapter 20).

• Chemical hot packs.

• A floating knife, a Swiss Army knife, a whetstone, and stainless steel eating utensils.

• Extra pine plugs to repair the raft.

• Plastic bags.

• Fishing tackle: hooks, lures, and sinkers in various sizes; 16-pound test monofilament line (200 yards); gang hook; a drop line; wire leaders; a gaff; and a spear gun.

• Signaling devices: four hand-held flares, three rocket or parachute flares, a mirror, a waterproof flashlight with signaling switch and spare batteries, a whistle, a hand-held VHF radio, and dye-markers.

• Navigational equipment: a sextant, a compass, and a watch with luminous dials; nautical charts (including a seasonal pilot's chart of the area); a copy of the *Nautical Almanac*; a set of sight reduction tables; a speed log; a log, pencils, pads of paper, and a pencil sharpener. (Store these items and the medical kit in a waterproof bag.)

This survival bag should be waterproof and buoyant. Store it in an accessible place so that it can be retrieved quickly in an emergency.

FIRST THINGS FIRST

Events can unfold with lightning speed when your boat hits a whale or a steel container in mid-ocean and starts to settle by the head. So Steven Callahan discovered when his sloop *Napoleon Solo* struck a mysterious object in the mid-Atlantic one night in 1984:

> BANG! A deafening explosion blankets the subtler sounds of torn wood fiber and rush of sea. I jump up. Water thunders over me as if I've suddenly been thrown into the path of a rampaging river. Forward, aft—where does it come from? Is half the side gone? No time. I fumble with the knife I have sheathed by the chart table. Already the water is waist deep. The nose of the boat is dipping down. Solo comes to a halt as she begins a sickening dive. She's going down, down!

When the water starts rising in the bilge, you've got to stay cool and think clearly. You'll go down with your ship if you and your crew don't maintain your composure, think clearly, and act decisively. Don't abandon ship unless you have no choice. But once you decide to take to the boats, these are your priorities.

Flotation

Put on your PFD (personal flotation device) at the first sign of trouble. If you can't get your survival craft launched before your boat sinks, and you have to go into the water, gather flotsam about you and hang onto it. (It will give you extra buoyancy, and some of it may be useful to you later.) Pull yourself as far out of the water as you can onto anything big enough to support you. If you aren't wearing a PFD, turn your trousers into an air bladder: Take them off and tie the ends of the legs together with a tight square knot. Then inflate them by swinging them over your head by the waist, or by holding them upside down underwater and blowing air into them.

First Aid

Once you and your crew get into the survival raft, check to see if anyone is injured. Stabilize the injured as well as you can. Control bleeding, splint fractures, and administer analgesics as appropriate. Perform CPR on any submersion victim who isn't breathing.

Signaling

The moment you realize you are going to take to the boats, turn on your EPIRB. It will broadcast a continuous signal for at least 48 hours on a distress frequency monitored by aircraft, ships, and satellites.

If you have time, issue a distress call. Tune your VHF radio to Channel 16, press the microphone button, and repeat: "Mayday! Mayday! Mayday!" Then, do the following.

• Say: "This is [boat name, radio call sign]." Repeat three times.
• Say: "Mayday. My position is _____."
• Say: "The boat is [describe condition of boat]."
• Say: "We require [describe what kind of assistance you need]."
• Say: "There are _____ adults and _____ children aboard with _____ injuries."
• Say: "[Boat name] is [length, type, color]."
• Say: "I will listen on Channel 16. This is [boat name and call sign]. Over."

Release the microphone button and monitor Channel 16. Repeat the message if there is no response. If you don't get a response after several transmissions, repeat the distress signal on any other VHF frequency you think might be heard.

If you are more than 20 miles off shore, first transmit your distress signal to a shore station over your SSB (single sideband) radio. Then, broadcast the message on Channel 16 in case any ships are in the area. Before you leave the vessel, lock the VHF transmitter on the air (on a channel other than 16) by taping down the microphone button. This will give rescuers a signal to home in on.

Also, if you have time, take a position fix and write it down so you won't forget it. Note the Loran, RDF, and radar bearings, when appropriate.

Rockets and flares may help you to attract the attention of passing ships at night. Parachute signals can be launched to a height of over 1,000 feet and can be seen for 35 to 40 miles on a clear night. Rockets can be seen up to 20 miles; flares up to 5 miles. Smoke signals and dye markers are more effective during the daytime. The flash of a signal mirror can be seen from altitudes as high as 35,000 feet. In fact, a pilot will see the flash before you see his aircraft, so flash your mirror in the direction of the sound of a plane even if you can't see it. If you know that a sea and air rescue attempt has been launched, flash the mirror continuously. It can't hurt to flash it toward the horizon whenever you think of it, even if you don't think that a rescue attempt is underway.

WATER

Water, water, every where,
And all the boards did shrink;
Water, water, every where,
Nor any drop to drink.

—Samuel Taylor Coleridge,
The Rime of the Ancient Mariner

You can survive for weeks without food, but only a few days without water. Drinking salt water is taboo. Its high mineral content will make you delirious and worsen your dehydration. And drinking urine is just as bad. It, too, is highly concentrated, and it is loaded with metabolic waste. Drinking urine will worsen dehydration.

Water Procurement

You should keep one or two 5-gallon water containers on deck ready to throw into your raft in an emergency. Fill them only three-quarters full so that they will float, and attach a 10-foot polypropylene tether so they can be towed if there is no room for them in the raft. Store several containers of distilled water in the raft also.

If time permits before abandoning ship, drink your fill of water. Once in the raft, don't ration water; drink to quench your thirst. It's essential that you maintain optimal strength and stamina for as long as possible, and depriving yourself of water is not the way to do it. The digestion and elimination of food increases your water requirement, so don't eat any food unless you have plenty of water. (You're much more likely to die of thirst than starvation. Your body will cannibalize itself, converting fat and protein in the tissues into glucose, and most of us have enough fat and muscle to stay alive for several weeks.)

After you get settled, rig up the solar stills. On sunny days, they each should yield about 48 ounces of fresh water. Be on the lookout for *rain,* and always have containers ready to collect as much rainwater as possible. You can use the roof of your canopy, boots, shoes, oil skins, sails, plastic bags, cans, and even fish or turtle intestines (tie a knot in one end, and turn it inside out). Make sure you rinse the containers in salt water first to dissolve accumulated salt. Then use the first few ounces to moisten your lips or clean yourself. When you've quenched your thirst and filled all your containers, take a shower, if the rainwater is warm. It'll give you a real shot in the arm. And make sure you use the rainwater first; stored water will stay fresh longer than rainwater.

If the days are warm and the nights are cold, *dew* will collect on surfaces exposed to air. Wipe it up with a rag, wring the rag out over a container, and drink the water.

If you are shipwrecked in cold waters, you can melt *old sea ice* and drink it. Old ice is blue, has rounded edges, and breaks easily into flakes.

Fish eyes contain fresh water; they are as sweet as grapes when you are half-crazed by thirst. After you have cleaned the flesh off any fish you might catch, snap the spine and suck out the *spinal fluid.* It contains fresh water, glucose, and protein. You can squeeze a few drops of potable fluid out of any fish or other marine life you catch with a juice press. If you don't have a press, you can section the fish, fold it up in a cloth, and squeeze the fluid out of the flesh by twisting the ends of the cloth. And you can carve holes in the side of a large fish and allow lymphatic fluid to accumulate in the holes.

Dougal Robertson and his family may not have survived their 37-day ordeal in the eastern Pacific had they not been able to quench their thirst with *turtle blood:*

> *I held the plastic cup under the copious flow of blood, the cup filled quickly . . . and then raising the full cup to my lips, [I] tested it cautiously. It wasn't salty at all! I tilted the cup and drained it. "Good stuff!" I shouted. I felt as if I had just consumed the elixir of life.*

> —Dougal Robertson,
> *Survive the Savage Sea*

Minimizing Water Losses

One way in which the body dissipates internal heat is through *evaporation* of sweat on the surface of the skin. In hot weather, you will lose 1.5 to 3.5 quarts of water each hour through evaporation. You can't sustain water losses like that for long without feeling like Coleridge's Ancient Mariner:

> *With throats unslaked, with black lips baked,*
> *We could nor laugh nor wail;*

You can limit evaporative heat loss on hot days by staying cool. Harness yourself to the raft and get into the water (keep a weather eye out for sharks!) or douse yourself with sea water periodically to keep your clothing wet. Partially deflate the bottom of your raft to decrease the insulating effect of the inflation chamber, and open the flaps to increase ventilation. Exert yourself as little as possible. If the seas are rough, take seasickness pills to avoid vomiting.

SHELTER

Clothing

Protective clothing can make life on a survival craft more bearable. Gather up some long pants, long-sleeved shirts, a hat, a bandanna, long underwear, oil skins, and a couple of pairs of white socks, and stow them in the raft before abandoning ship.

Raft

Don't inflate your raft until you're ready to get into it, and launch it from the lee side. If the boat is listing heavily, enter the raft from the high side so you won't be dragged under if the boat capsizes. Take off your shoes, and remove sharp objects from your pockets. If you reboard the sinking vessel, tie up alongside with a long painter, and carry a sharp knife with you so you can cut it if the boat suddenly goes under.

If you abandon ship in *warm waters*, erect the canopy and partially deflate the floor. Protect yourself from sunburn by wearing protective clothing, sunscreen, and a physical sun block on your nose, ears, cheeks, and lips.

In *cold waters*, erect the canopy or set up a windscreen. Change to dry clothing whenever you get a dousing, and wear a hat and as much insulating clothing as possible. Cover the floor with blankets or cloth to retard heat loss, and huddle in the center of the raft with your raftmates. Wiggle your fingers and toes periodically to maintain circulation and ward off frostbite. If water supplies are ample, eat frequently.

Inflatable life rafts are durable if you steer clear of lovesick swordfish. Maurice and Maraly Bailey survived 119 days in the eastern Pacific in an inflatable raft, and Steve Callahan's raft held together long enough for him to make a landfall on Guadeloupe after drifting across the Atlantic for 76 days. To keep the raft seaworthy:

• Inspect the skin daily for chafing, particularly around the flaps and handles, where towing lines, drogue lines, and grab lines attach, and at the angle formed by the floor and walls of the raft. Lines that are chafing the fabric of the raft should be wrapped with cloth.

• Set out a baffle sheet made up of extra sails or clothing to prevent fish from bumping against the sides and bottom of the raft.

• Ward off sharks and lovesick turtles with a sharp rap on the snout with an oar or paddle.

• Repair leaks in the inflation chambers immediately.

• Carefully stow knives, fishhooks, and other sharp objects.

• Don't overinflate the chambers, and release some air on hot days so they don't overexpand.

• Keep vital equipment secured when not in use so that you don't lose it if the raft capsizes. Don't stand in the raft. Have the heaviest people sit in the center, and avoid sudden movements.

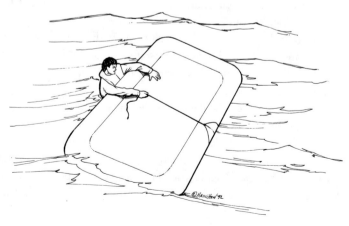

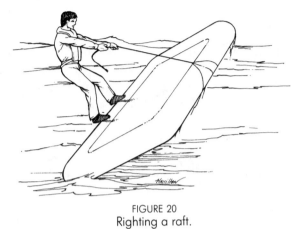

FIGURE 20
Righting a raft.

Use the sea anchor as needed in heavy seas. If the raft cap-sizes, throw the righting rope across the bottom, move to the opposite side of the raft, brace your foot on the edge of the raft, and pull on the rope. The raft will flip right over (see Figure 20).

FOOD

There are no finicky eaters in a life raft. Magellan's crew was reduced at one point to eating biscuit that was "but a powder full of worms, and in addition it was stinking with the urine of rats." They also ate the hide that covered the main yard, sawdust, and rats (which they considered a delicacy). The annals of the sea are replete with stories of cannibalism.

> For a month we'd neither wittles nor drink,
> Till a-hungry we did feel,
> So we drawed a lot, and accordin' shot
> The captain for our meal.
>
> —Sir William S. Gilbert,
> *The Yarn of the Nancy Bell*

Fish

If you find yourself hungrily eyeing your raftmates, it's time you caught some fish. If you don't have a fishing kit on board, improvise. You can unravel strands of canvas or cloth to make a few feet of line. You can use a bent nail or an open safety pin as a hook, or fashion hooks out of scraps of wood. First, whittle a 2- to 3-inch-long shaft, and cut a notch in one end. Then, seat a 1- to 2-inch-long point or a fish bone in this notch at a 30-degree angle to the shaft, and secure it to the shaft with string. Make sure the point is hard and sharp (see Figure 21).

Here's a fiendishly clever way to catch fish: Sharpen both ends of a short piece of wood or bone, tie your line to the middle of it, and insert it lengthwise into a piece of bait. When a fish tugs on it, give it a short yank to pull it crossways and bury the sharp ends into his flesh.

Fish and bird entrails make excellent bait, or you can net min-

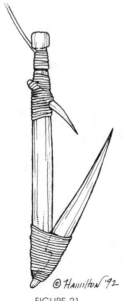

FIGURE 21
Wooden fishhooks.

nows with a towel. Cut a long, thin piece of fish skin and attach it and a silver-dollar-sized hunk of bird or fish flesh to your hook. If your raft is drifting at a decent speed, let out 30 or 40 feet of line and trail it in the wake. Or you can try *jigging*. Attach a sinker to the end of the line, and then repeatedly raise the line up and down through an excursion of ten feet or so until you hook a fish.

A sure-fire angling technique is to hook a minnow or another small fish through the lips or dorsal fin and let him swim around until he is eaten by a larger fish. Then, set the hook, play the fish until he's exhausted, and pull him in. You can also cut off one of the minnow's lateral fins so that he can't swim straight. He'll flop on the surface of the water until a predator fish detects the abnormal vibrations and moves in for the kill.

You can make *lures* out of shiny metal, buttons, coins, fish skin, bird feathers, or brightly colored cloth. On a bright, moonlit night, you can attract fish by reflecting moonshine onto the water near your raft.

The most productive way to catch fish is with a *spear gun*. If you don't have one, fashion a spear out of a wooden paddle. Carve at least one sharp barb into the business end of the spear, and attach a wrist loop to the other end so a speared fish doesn't yank the spear out of your hands and swim off with it.

Diving birds indicate areas where large fish are feeding on schools of smaller fish. Cast a lure into the water where the birds are diving and retrieve it quickly, or use a gang hook to snare fish.

As you drift along, your raft will become a marine ecosystem. Plants and barnacles growing on the bottom of the raft will attract schools of fish, and you should have luck fishing in the shadow cast by the raft. You should also do well at night when fish come to the surface to feed. Try to attract flying fish into your raft with a flashlight or a mirror reflecting moonlight.

Most pelagic fish (those living in the open sea) are edible. The heart, liver, and blood are especially nourishing, but you'd be wise to cook the intestines before eating them. You may find a few partially digested fish when you slit open the belly of a large fish. Fish flesh rapidly deteriorates, so eat what you can quickly. Then cut the remainder into strips and leave them in the sun to dry.

Seaweed

Your raft will grow a beard of seaweed after a few days. Seaweed is very salty and unappetizing, but it's a rich source of shrimp, crabs, and other forms of edible marine life.

Birds

"God save thee, ancient Mariner!
From the fiends, that plague thee thus!—
Why look'st thou so?"—With my cross-bow
I shot the ALBATROSS.

The Ancient Mariner and his shipmates paid a terrible price for his indiscretion. Sailors once ascribed mystical powers to sea birds. Many believed that gulls were the wandering spirits of drowned sailors and harming a sea bird would bring bad luck.

Whether you're superstitious or not, if you're starving, a Mother Carey's chicken, tern, or booby will look as appetizing as pheasant under glass. All sea birds are edible, and you can catch them by trolling a baited fishhook or a sharp-edged, triangular, baited piece of metal. The hook or metal will catch in the bird's mouth, and you can pull him in like a fish. If a booby alights on your raft, grab him. If he is wary, tie two pieces of line together in a loose knot, and tie two of the free ends to the raft. Then put some bait inside the loop. When a booby starts eating the bait, pull the knot tight around his legs. (Now you know why they're called "boobies"!)

NAVIGATION

Captain William Bligh wasn't the most popular skipper, but he was a world-class navigator and small-boat handler. After the crew of the *Bounty* mutinied, they put him and seventeen of his officers into an open, 23-foot launch with a little bread and water, a compass, and a sextant (but no charts) and set them adrift near Tafua, east of the Fiji Islands. In a brilliant display of seamanship, Bligh navigated the launch 3,618 nautical miles to the Dutch Island of Timor, north of Australia.

The modern inflatable life raft is not designed for a voyage like Bligh's. Its function is to keep you alive until you are rescued by SAR (search and rescue) craft. If you transmitted a distress signal before you abandoned ship, you'd be wise to remain in the area where your vessel went down. If help doesn't arrive within 24 hours, however, you may want to strike out for a shipping lane or land. To make a rational decision on whether to stay or go, you must consider such factors as:

- Whether your craft can be sailed or rowed.
- Your food and water supplies.
- Your physical condition and the condition of the raft.
- Your navigational skills, and whether you have the necessary instruments and charts.
- The distance to land or shipping lanes.

If your raft isn't well stocked with food, water, and equipment, and you aren't confident in your navigational skills, slow your drift with a drogue and wait for rescuers to show up.

If you decide to go for it, study charts of the area and determine what your most likely landfall will be, based on prevailing winds and currents. Ideally, you should aim for a busy shipping lane with a large land mass or island chain downwind and downcurrent from it, in case you aren't rescued by a ship.

Navigational Techniques

The goddess Juno gave Jason a talking oak figurehead for his ship, the *Argo,* and he consulted it frequently as he navigated the *Argo* across the Mediterranean in his search for the Golden Fleece. If your raft doesn't have a talking figurehead, you'll have to fix your position each day and plot it on a chart. If navigation is not your strong suit, follow these steps to determine latitude and longitude.

Determine Latitude

1. Use your sextant to take an altitude observation of Polaris, or the Southern Cross if you are in the southern hemisphere. (If you don't have a sextant, either a protractor, a compass rose, or a piece of plotting paper will suffice.) The altitude of Polaris equals your latitude to within a degree or two. You can use tables in the *Nautical Almanac* to correct your reading to the nearest half degree of latitude (30 miles).

2. Take an altitude of the sun or any star or planet whose *declination* (position north or south of the equator) at median transit (when it passes over your meridian, i.e., noon) is listed in the *Nautical Almanac*. Then add or subtract the zenith distance (90 degrees minus the observed altitude) to the declination to find the latitude (see Figure 22).

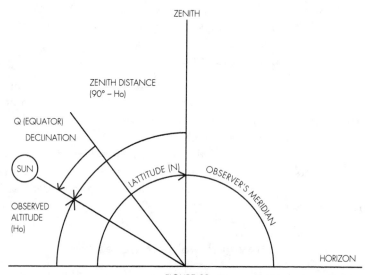

FIGURE 22
Determining latitude: latitude = declination $+/-$ zenith distance (here the observer is in northern latitudes with the sun in southerly declination at median transit).

From *How to Survive on Land and Sea*, 4th Edition, by Frank C. Craighead, Jr. and John J. Craighead; Revised by Ray E. Smith and D. Shiras Jarvis. Copyright © 1984 by the U.S. Naval Institute, Annapolis, Maryland.

Determine Longitude

The sun travels east to west at the rate of 15 degrees of longitude per hour. You can use this fact to calculate longitude. Set your watch to Greenwich Mean Time (GMT), and record the GMT of the median transit of the sun. (You can do this by marking the exact GMT when a due northerly or southerly shadow is cast by a stick attached to your canopy.) Then read off the meridian transit at Greenwich from the *equation of time* in the *Nautical Almanac*. To calculate your longitude, subtract the GMT of meridian transit at Greenwich from the exact GMT of meridian transit at your position. Then convert this time difference to an arc difference. You can look this up in the arc/time conversion table in the *Nautical Almanac*, or simply multiply the time difference by 15. If the GMT local noon is later than GMT noon Greenwich, the longitude is *westerly*. If it is earlier, the longitude is *easterly*.

Longitude =
(GMT local noon − GMT noon Greenwich) × 15 degrees/hour

Dead Reckoning

You should also plot a *dead-reckoning* track. Dead reckoning is the determination of a boat's position based on the course steered (direction of drift, in the case of a raft) and speed through the water since its last accurately determined position. Determine direction with a magnetic compass. Then find the variation for your locale on your nautical chart, and *add* westerly variation and *subtract* easterly variation to find the true course. (Just remember, "East is least, and west is best.")

If you don't have a compass, observe the prevailing wave pattern and its relationship to the sun, which is due north or south at noon. At night, note the relationship of the wave pattern to Polaris, which bears roughly due north, or the Southern Cross, which bears due south.

Trail a log to determine your speed through the water.

MAKING A LANDFALL

The dawn showed us a storm-torn ocean, and the morning passed without bringing us a sight of the land; but at 1 P.M., through a rift in the flying mists, we got a glimpse of the huge crags of the island and realized that our position had become desperate. We were on a dead lee shore, and we could gauge our approach to the unseen cliffs by the roar of the breakers against the sheer walls of rock.

—Sir Ernest Shackleton, *South*

Getting ground to pulp by waves breaking on a rocky shore takes all the fun out of a landfall. But if you can detect signs of land, you may be able to avoid a smashing conclusion to your voyage. (Lee shores were the least of Jason's worries. On his voyage to find the Golden Fleece, he had to navigate the *Argo* around the treacherous Wandering Rocks, which would crash together whenever a ship tried to pass between them.)

Mariners of old could "smell" land long before it came into view. Your olfactory sense may not be that acute, but if you watch for these signs of land, you'll have plenty of time to guide your raft to a safe landfall.

Clouds

Stationary clouds indicate an underlying land mass beyond the horizon. Fixed cumulus clouds often hover over mountainous or high land. A bright aura on the horizon may be caused by sunlight reflected off a sandy beach, ice- or snow-covered land, or shallow water. Sunlight reflected off the shallow water of a coral reef causes lagoon glare, a green tint in the sky or under a cloud.

Water Color

The deeper the water, the bluer it is. As the water becomes shallower, it turns lighter shades of green. Brown or black areas indicate coral shoals.

Floating Debris

Floating vegetation, driftwood, and human refuse are reliable signs that land is near.

Birds

Sailors' esteem for birds seems to have no bounds. Some even believe having a bird defecate on them brings good luck. You can put stock in that if you want to, but don't rely on birds to estimate your proximity to land. The variety of species and number of birds will increase as you draw nearer to land, but shore birds are often seen hundreds of miles from land, and land birds can be blown far out to sea by storms. On the other hand, many a mariner has been warned off a rocky shore in thick weather by the crying of gulls.

SUMMARY OF ABANDON-SHIP PROCEDURES

1. Put on PFDs.
2. Transmit a distress signal.
3. Turn on the EPIRB.
4. Try to save the boat.
5. Bring the survival bag on deck.
6. Gather as much food from the galley as possible.
7. Drink your fill of water.
8. Take a position fix.
9. Launch the raft and load the survival bag, water cans, food, and passengers.

If your boat is sinking *fast*, streamline the procedure:

1. Don PFDs.
2. Send a distress signal.
3. Launch the raft.
4. Grab the survival bag and water cans and get into the raft.

After you get into the raft, it's important that one person assume command and oversee the following procedures:

1. Paddle away from the sinking boat.
2. Set out the drogue.
3. Make sure the raft is fully inflated.
4. Pull swimmers into the raft.
5. Tether rafts, if there is more than one.

6. Attend to the sick or injured.
7. Turn on the EPIRB.
8. Retrieve usable flotsam, e.g., sails, spars, and oars.
9. Establish seating arrangements.
10. Tie the equipment to the sides of the raft.
11. Establish a watch schedule.
12. Start a log.
13. Set up solar stills.
14. Study charts, become familiar with prevailing winds and currents, and estimate the most likely landfall.

As day succeeds monotonous day, and the sun blisters your body and scorches your soul, your spirits will sag. Just remember the words of Dougal Robertson who, after failing to attract the attention of a passing ship, fought back from the edge of despair to lead his family to salvation after 38 days at sea in a dinghy:

> I surveyed the empty flare cartons bitterly, and the one smoke flare which was damp and wouldn't work, and something happened to me in that instant, that for me changed the whole aspect of our predicament. If these poor bloody seamen couldn't rescue us, then we would have to make it on our own and to hell with them. We would survive without them, yes, and that was the word from now on, "survival," not "rescue," or "help," or dependence of any kind, just survival. I felt the strength flooding through me, lifting me from the depression of disappointment to a state of almost cheerful abandon. I felt the bitter aggression of the predator fill my mind. . . . We would live for three months or six months from the sea if necessary. . . . From that instant on I became a savage.

12
SEASICKNESS

Harvey staggered over the wet decks to the nearest rail. He was very unhappy; but he saw the deck steward lashing chairs together, and, since he had boasted before the man that he was never seasick, his pride made him go aft to the second-saloon deck at the stern. . . . The deck was deserted, and he crawled to the extreme end of it. . . . There he doubled up in limp agony, for the Wheeling "stogie" joined with the surge and jar of the screw to sieve out his soul. His head swelled; sparks of fire danced before his eyes; his body seemed to lose weight, while his heels wavered in the breeze. He was fainting from seasickness, and a roll of the ship tilted him over the rail. . . . Then a low, gray mother-wave swung out of the fog, tucked Harvey under one arm . . . and pulled him off and away to leeward; the great green closed over him, and he went quietly to sleep.

—Rudyard Kipling, *Captains Courageous*

Anyone can get seasick is if the conditions are bad enough. Tell me Captain Queeg didn't get a little green around the gills when the *Caine* was being tossed around like a cork in that Pacific typhoon. Sure, Nelson was made a lord after crushing the French fleet in the battle of the Nile, but I'll bet there were times when he would have traded his peerage for a bottle of Dramamine. And even that crusty old sea dog Captain Ahab must have had days when he would have given his right leg for a scopolamine patch.

Seasickness is the pits. I know. I worked as a deck hand on an oil tanker one summer when I was in college, and I learned first-hand what a miserable affliction it can be. We were steaming north past Cape Hatteras when a hurricane roared up out of the Caribbean and hit us from behind like a mugger with a crowbar. It was like a scene from *Victory at Sea:* Seventy-knot winds whipped the sea into a foaming, frothing frenzy. Mountainous waves slammed into the ship, knocking her about like a toy boat, each one threatening to stove in her plates and send her to the bottom.

I remember the scene because I had a front-row seat out on the catwalk that connected the fore and aft sections of the ship. I was in danger of being washed overboard, but I clung to my precarious perch like a cat in a tree. All that rolling and lurching had made me seasick, and I felt better on the catwalk because it was in the center of the ship, where motion was minimal. I stayed out there in the wind and rain for hours until, finally, the bosun lured me back inside with the promise of a cure for my seasickness. I envisioned some elixir, passed down from one generation of old salts to the next, a magic potion that would put me out of my misery.

The bosun sat me down at a table and put a bowl of piping hot stewed tomatoes in front of me. I devoured them hungrily, taking it on faith that they would cure my seasickness. And they did.

Now, there's nothing magical about stewed tomatoes. They have no more medicinal value than such traditional folk cures as creosote, horseradish and red herrings, salt water, pickles, dried fish, diesel oil and fish guts, or salt pork (tied to a string, swallowed, and retrieved after 5 minutes). But mariners have been curing seasickness with rotgut concoctions like these since the first caveman set out in a dugout canoe. The success of these supposed cures is the result of the *placebo effect:* the "medicine" makes you better because you believe it will.

MOTION COMMOTION

That's not to say that seasickness is all in your head. Seasickness is a real problem. A data processing problem. We have three systems that receive and process raw information about our posture and orientation in space. These stabilizing systems are:

1. The *visual system,* the eyes and their nerve connections to the brain.

2. A system of *position and pressure sensors* in the muscles, skin, and joints.

3. The *vestibular system*. This consists of three *semicircular canals* and an *otolithic apparatus* in each inner ear, as well as their nerve connections to the brain. The semicircular canals sense angular acceleration (spinning and turning motion), while the otolithic apparatus senses linear acceleration (straight-ahead motion), as well as static gravitational forces.

These three systems work together to keep you on an even keel. As long as there is a smooth, steady flow of concordant information from each of the three systems, everything is copacetic. The systems function fine when you're skimming across Lake George in your vintage Century runabout on a glorious summer day and the surface is smooth as glass. But come back to do a little salmon fishing in late October and it's a different story. The waves will be 5 feet high, your boat will be rocking and rolling, and you'll be running around like a one-armed paperhanger, trying to run those downriggers with one hand and drive the boat with the other. Under conditions like that, the brain is hit with a stream of discordant information from the three stabilizing systems. Your eyes may be looking at the motion of the waves, but your inner ear and body-position sensors detect the motion of the heaving deck. When these conflicting sensory reports reach the brain, the circuits become overloaded, and the vomiting center in the brain is activated. The next thing you know, you're hanging your head over the side.

> For sheer downright misery give me a hurricane, not too warm, the yard of a sailing ship, a wet sail and a bout of sea-sickness.
>
> —Apsley Cherry-Garrard, *The Worst Journey in the World*

SYMPTOMS

Your first clue that you're going to be seasick is a cold sweat. You may also get a mild headache, feel a little drowsy, and start yawning or hyperventilating. You may turn a little green around the gills, and then become profoundly nauseated. (It's no coincidence that *naus*, the root for *nausea*, means "ship" in Greek.) When you start to drool like a rabid dog, you know that your next stop is the rail.

GETTING YOUR SEA LEGS

You *can* get used to rough seas and a heaving deck. After a few days at sea, your brain begins to filter out some of the information coming in from the eyes, joints, muscles, and ears, retaining just enough to allow you to keep your balance and not get seasick. It's called "habituation," or "getting your sea legs." Most blue-water sailors habituate after a day or two at sea. Unfortunately, habituation is not forever. If you go ashore for a couple of days, you will have to rehabituate when you go back out to sea. But the brain retains a memory of the pattern of motion, so you'll get your sea legs back quickly.

Prevention
No one is immune to seasickness. Even the crusty old salts who sailed the tea packets around the Horn became seasick when the seas got high enough. *When* you get seasick depends on your basic susceptibility, the severity of the stimulus (how rough is the sea?), and the duration of the stimulus. If the sea is rough enough for long enough, everyone on board will get seasick.

Fortunately, there are a number of preventative techniques and medications you can use to avoid *mal de mer*. Here are some tricks that have stood the test of time.

• *Maintain a steady gaze on the horizon* or a stationary object, such as an island, a lighthouse, or the shoreline. With a fixed point to focus on, the brain has a steady visual reference by which to judge sensory signals from the ears and the body-position sensors.

• *Stay topside.* Don't make the classic mistake of going into the cabin to lie down. There's no fixed object that you can focus on in a cabin, so your seasickness will worsen. And stale cabin air is no help at all.

• *Avoid unpleasant smells, loud noises, and vibration.* Any strong sensory stimulus can aggravate seasickness. Stay away from the stern, especially if the boat is powered by an outboard motor. And steer clear of the bait box.

• *Stay amidships,* where there is less movement. Stay on your feet, and roll with the boat.

• *Keep your mind occupied.* If you start to feel sick, dwelling on it will only make matters worse. Maintain a running conversation with your shipmates, crack jokes, or recite poetry to get your mind off the heaving, rolling motion of the boat.

• *Placebos.* Eat a bowl of stewed tomatoes if you start to feel sick. Or Chinese apples, if you think they'll help. Anxiety and stress play a big role in seasickness, and a placebo can be a powerful tool in preventing illness. If you don't have a cast-iron stomach, it's best to stick to a liquid diet starting the morning of your trip, with no solids at all until you've got your sea legs.

• *Stay well-hydrated and well-rested.* Dehydration and fatigue reduce your threshold for seasickness. Life-raft survivors, who often are extremely tired and dehydrated, have severe problems with seasickness.

• *Refrain from alcohol,* at least during the first stage of your voyage. An alcohol-fogged brain takes longer to adapt to sensory overload and conflict.

The Medicine Chest

There are a number of medications that can prevent seasickness. You'd be smart to keep some of these preparations in your ship's medicine chest for a stormy day.

• *Meclizine* (Antivert). An antihistamine effective in preventing or treating seasickness. Take 25 to 50 mg 1 hour before setting out on the water, and repeat the dose every 24 hours.

• *Diphenhydramine* (Benadryl). Take 25 to 50 mg 2 hours before you weigh anchor and repeat every 6 hours, as needed. Diphenhydramine has a potent soporific effect, so if it's your turn at the wheel and you're in a busy shipping lane, use something else.

• *Dimenhydrinate* (Dramamine). A tried-and-true seasickness remedy that is effective in preventing and treating *mal de mer*. Drowsiness is its main drawback.

• *Promethazine* (Phenergan). A prescription antihistamine that you can use to prevent seasickness or treat its symptoms. It is a potent antiemetic and sedative. Available in oral, suppository, and injectable form.

• *Ephedrine.* A great drug for treating seasickness once it starts. The dose is 25 to 50 mg initially, and 25 mg every 3 to 4 hours as needed. (Ephedrine is a stimulant and may cause insomnia.)

• *Scopolamine* (Transderm Scōp). A patch worn behind the ear that releases a steady stream of scopolamine into the bloodstream. Put on a patch the night before your trip, and you won't have to worry about seasickness for three days. However, you may get dry mouth, blurred vision, drowsiness, impaired short-term memory, or toxic psychosis (an infrequent adverse reaction to scopolamine consisting of hallucinations, disorientation, amnesia, and confusion). You can also get a *withdrawal syndrome* from scopolamine patches after using them. The symptoms include dizziness, nausea, vomiting, headache, and loss of balance. Scopolamine is a prescription drug and is contraindicated in anyone with a history of glaucoma.

I recommend that you use meclizine to prevent seasickness. If you get sick despite the meclizine, a 50-mg Phenergan suppository will usually cure your *mal de mer*.

You should avail yourself of any technique or medicine you think may control seasickness, but keep in mind the old English sailors' proverb: "The only cure for seasickness is to sit on the shady side of an old brick church in the country."

.
.
.
.
.

13

SUNBURN AND
OTHER SOLAR INJURIES

O sun!
Burn the great sphere thou mov'st in; darkling
Stand
The varying shores o' the world.

—William Shakespeare, *Antony and Cleopatra*

Everyone has his own conception of hell. The biblical lake of fire, an eternity on Devil's Island, or hours spent locked in a small room with one's mother-in-law all hold special horrors for some people. Personally, I can think of nothing more hellish than to be shipwrecked on a tropical sea—drifting aimlessly in an open boat, pushed this way and that by wind and tide, never again to walk on solid ground or see another human face. Seasickness, thirst, and loneliness I could probably handle. The thought of sharks circling my boat, closing in for a human repast, though not a pleasant prospect, doesn't overly disturb me. What does strike fear in my heart is the thought of lying out there in the open, day after endless day, unprotected from the ravages of the sun, my skin baking in the ultraviolet rays.

Boaters everywhere, whether they are languishing in a lifeboat or tooling around Puget Sound in a runabout, are vulnerable to the acute and chronic effects of exposure to the sun. Every minute you are out in the sun you are bombarded with radiation from all across the electromagnetic spectrum, everything from cosmic, gamma, and X rays to microwaves and ultraviolet and infrared waves. Infrared rays and microwaves may not hurt you, but ultraviolet rays will fry your epidermis.

THE ELECTROMAGNETIC SPECTRUM

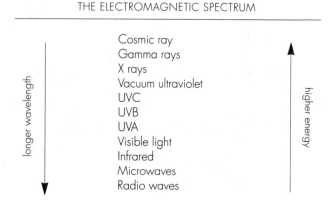

Cosmic ray
Gamma rays
X rays
Vacuum ultraviolet
UVC
UVB
UVA
Visible light
Infrared
Microwaves
Radio waves

longer wavelength

higher energy

ULTRAVIOLET RADIATION

Ultraviolet radiation (UVR) comes in three varieties: ultraviolet A (UVA, wavelength 320 to 400 nm), ultraviolet B (UVB, wavelength 290 to 320 nm), and ultraviolet C (UVC, wavelength 200 to 290 nm). The ozone layer absorbs UVC, but most UVA and UVB rays penetrate the ozone shield and strike the earth's surface. That's bad news for boaters, because UVB causes sunburn, premature aging, and skin cancer, and UVA exposure leads to "sun cataracts" and sun allergies.

THE SKINNY ON SKIN

Your tolerance for UVR is genetically determined and depends on your skin type (see the table on page 165), which is a function of how much melanin you have in your epidermis. Melanin is the dark pigment that causes tanning and blocks transmission of UVR into the deeper layers of the skin. If you are a blonde or a redhead of Celtic extraction, with blue or green eyes, then you have only a smattering of melanin in your epidermis. You could be staked out on the beach for the entire month of August and you wouldn't tan. However, you would get a memorable sunburn. If you are of Mediterranean or Latin American descent, and have dark hair

SKIN TYPE	BURNING/TANNING CHARACTERISTICS	EXAMPLES
I	Always burns, never tans	Blonds and red-heads, blue eyes
II	Usually burns, tans after many hours in the sun	Fair-skinned, blondes
III	Burns and tans moderately	Most Caucasians
IV	Burns slightly, tans well	Hispanics and Asians
V	Almost never burns, tans darkly	Middle Easterners, Asian Indians, Native Americans
VI	Burns only with very heavy exposure	Blacks, Africans, African Americans

and brown eyes, you have a relative abundance of melanin in your epidermis, tan easily, and rarely burn.

LEARNING THE ANGLES

You can't switch skins, but you can control some of the other factors that determine your exposure to UVR. Many of these factors are a function of the *solar zenith angle*, which is the angle at which the sun's rays strike the earth's surface. The greater the solar zenith angle, the less distance sunlight has to travel through the atmosphere, and the more UVR gets through. The solar zenith angle in turn is determined by the time of day, time of year, and latitude.

High noon is the most dangerous time to be out in the sun because the sun is at its zenith then and its rays have to travel a shorter distance through the atmosphere before striking your skin. Eighty percent of the sunburn- and cancer-causing UVB rays strike the earth's surface between 9 A.M. and 3 P.M., and that's when you are at greatest risk for solar injury. UVA levels, on the other hand, remain almost uniform throughout the day.

You don't have to worry much about sunburn during the winter months, because the sun traverses a more southerly route across the sky. Even though the sun is closer to the earth, its intensity is decreased because it is low in the sky.

Latitude is an important determinant of sun exposure. Sunlight strikes the earth perpendicularly at the equator, and at progressively more oblique angles north and south of the equator. The sun's intensity decreases as you travel away from the equator and, as you might expect, so does the incidence of skin cancer.

Altitude is an important factor to keep in mind if you do your boating on fresh water. If you spend the day water-skiing on Lake Tahoe, you will be exposed to about 30 percent more UVR than you would on the same day at sea level. That's because Lake Tahoe is 6,229 feet above sea level, and the intensity of the sun's rays increases 4 to 5 percent with each 1,000-foot increase in elevation. The atmosphere is thinner at higher altitudes, and there is less smoke, dust, and water vapor to filter UVR.

Atmospheric conditions are an important part of the sun-exposure equation. Smoke and other air pollutants absorb UVR, while dust and water scatter it. Don't let your guard down on those cool, overcast summer days. Although heat-carrying infrared rays don't penetrate dense cloud cover, about 60 to 80 percent of UVR rays do. Just because it isn't warm and sunny doesn't mean there is no danger of sunburn. You can get badly burned if you don't cover up. And don't rely on your Bimini cover to protect you from the sun on overcast days. The haze bends the sun's rays and reflects them into shady areas. (Glass blocks transmission of UVB, so you *will* get some protection from your windshield.)

Surface conditions are important too. Sunlight is reflected by water, and choppy water reflects up to 100 percent of incident UVR. Wind alone can't cause a burn, but it can work in tandem with the sun to cause *windburn*. Wind dries and irritates sunburned skin, and by accelerating the evaporation of sweat it depletes the skin of urocanic acid, a UVR-screening chemical in the epidermis. And the cooling effect of the wind may lead you to spend more time in the sun then you should.

ASSESSING THE DAMAGES

If you play in the sun, you pay. Here are the penalties for excessive sun exposure.

Sunburn

Sunburn is an intense inflammatory response to UVR. The skin's first reaction to sun exposure is a transient reddening triggered by UVA. Then UVB gets into the act and causes a true sunburn reaction: redness, itching, and exquisite pain starting 2 to 8 hours after sun exposure and peaking in 24 to 36 hours. As in any partial-thickness burn, the skin may swell, blister, and slough. The redness fades over a period of 1 to 4 days, and the outermost layer of skin thickens and peels. Moist skin, high humidity, heat, and wind are all aggravating factors. If you really get fried over a large portion of your skin surface, you may experience vomiting, weakness, headache, chills, and fever, an illness quaintly described as "sun poisoning."

Photosensitivity

Sometimes the sun and certain chemicals, called "photosensitizers," can gang up on you to cause a *photosensitivity reaction*. These reactions can take one of three forms.

1. *Phototoxic reactions* are exaggerated sunburns triggered by UVA, and sometimes UVB, after the victim is exposed to a sensitizing chemical. These reactions are quite common and are often caused by perfumes, shampoos, and other frequently used products. A normal sunburn reaches its peak intensity 24 to 36 hours after exposure, but a phototoxic reaction continues to worsen over a period of 2 to 4 days. Individuals with skin types I or II are more likely to be prone to phototoxic reactions.

2. *Photoallergic reactions*, which are much less common, are eczema-like rashes triggered by exposure to UVA after the victim is sensitized by the chemicals in soaps, cosmetics, medications, or other products. Photoallergic reactions are equally common in people of all skin types, can be provoked by exposure to small amounts of UVR, and often affect areas of the skin not exposed to the sun.

3. *Phytophotodermatitis* is a phototoxic or photoallergic reaction mediated by skin exposure to a plant. Lemons, limes, celery, parsnip, parsley, fennel, dill, carrots, figs, mustard, and lichens are some of the common perpetrators of phytophotodermatitis. Spill a little lemon juice on your arm or leg at lunch, and that afternoon you may develop a severe sunburn or eczema-type reaction in the area after going out in the sun.

If you think you have been the victim of a photosensitivity reaction, you won't have to look far to find the culprit. Common photosensitizers include food additives (cyclamates and saccharine), shaving creams, after-shave lotions, certain tranquilizers, oral diabetes medications, diuretics, sulfa and tetracycline antibiotics, benzocaine, green soap, and even sunscreens.

Polymorphous Light Eruption

If you tend to get itchy bumps on your face and neck early every spring after your first day out in your boat, you probably *have* had PLE (polymorphous light eruption). Not to worry, though. After you have been out in the sun a few times, your skin "hardens" (thickens and tans) and the rash will go away. No one knows what causes PLE, but you can prevent it by covering up when you go out in the sun. And you can speed healing by applying a thin layer of 1% hydrocortisone ointment to the rash twice a day.

Skin Cancer

Scientists are predicting a worldwide epidemic of skin cancer in the coming years if current trends continue. The sun causes more than 95 percent of skin cancers, so boating enthusiasts are at high risk. I recommend an annual visit to your dermatologist to have your skin checked for these skin lesions.

1. *Actinic keratoses.* These are precancerous thickenings on the face, neck, and hands. Fifty percent of white people over age 40 have them. They should be removed before they degenerate into cancer.

2. *Basal cell carcinoma,* the most common skin cancer, is a painless, smooth, waxy thickening of the skin, usually found on the head and neck. These tumors rarely metastasize, but if ignored, they can kill by invading deep tissues.

3. *Squamous cell carcinoma* is a painless, crusty, red nodule with scales. It's usually seen on sun-exposed areas of the face and scalp. Early treatment can cure it.

4. *Malignant melanoma,* the infamous "black mole," is usually seen in people with fair skin, especially those who have had severe blistering sunburns. The incidence of malignant melanoma has doubled in the last decade, and it is predicted that the lifetime risk for white Americans will be 1 in 90 by the year 2000. If discovered early, malignant melanoma is curable. Use the ABCDs to distinguish melanoma from benign moles:

    a. Asymmetry—melanomas are asymmetric.

    b. Border—melanomas have irregular borders.

    c. Color—melanomas are different shades of blue, black, and brown.

    d. Diameter—melanomas are usually larger than a pencil eraser.

Sun Gets in Your Eyes

The only tissues in the body that sunburn are the skin and the eyes. These are some of the eye problems UVR can cause.

Photokeratitis

Do you remember the scenes in those old adventure movies where the mountain climber develops snow blindness and gets lost in the Alps or the Himalayas? Well, how would you like to get snow blindness while rounding Cape Horn in your sloop? You *can* get "snow blindness" when you're out on the water. Its medical name is *photokeratitis,* and it's a form of sunburn caused by

UVB rays reflecting off the surface of the water and striking your corneas.

You're a setup for photokeratitis when you cruise on unsettled, choppy waters on a bright, sunny day without wearing sunglasses or a hat. (Remember, choppy water can reflect up to 100 percent of the UVR waves that strike its surface.) Corneal UVR burns are painless at first. But 4 to 12 hours after exposure, you'll suddenly feel as though the wind blew hot cinders in your eyes. You'll have intense photophobia (fear of light), your eyelids will go into spasm, and the tears will flow like your bilge discharge.

Treatment

Have the ship's "doctor" instill one drop of 2% homatropine in each eye and then apply snug double patches. Rest in a dark cabin, apply cool compresses, and use analgesics as needed. Leave the patches on for 12 to 24 hours, and then make a promise to yourself never to go out in the sun without wearing a good pair of UVR-blocking sunglasses with side panels and a hat with a long brim.

Cataracts

Chronic exposure to UVR is associated with cataracts (opacification of the lens). UVB is the culprit, but it can be blocked by wearing eyeglasses that have been "dipped-coated" so that they are opaque to UVR or good-quality sunglasses that bar transmission of UVR. If nothing else, wearing a hat with a long brim will reduce eye exposure to UVR by 50 percent.

Solar Retinitis

Solar retinitis is a UVR-induced retinal injury caused by looking at the sun with binoculars or during a solar eclipse. The lens acts as a magnifying glass and focuses an intense beam of UVR on the *macula*, the area of the retina responsible for central vision. UVR can actually burn a small hole in the retina in this area, causing permanent central blindness (only peripheral vision remains).

Macular Degeneration

Macular degeneration, which causes legal blindness in 28 percent of Americans over age 75, *may* be related to chronic exposure to UVR. Another good reason to wear sunglasses.

PREVENTING SOLAR INJURY

The only sure way to avoid sun-damaged skin is to trade in your cabin cruiser for a submarine. If you can't swing that, then use some of these other tactics to avoid UVR bombardment.

1. *Avoid the midday sun*—the hours between 10 A.M. and 3 P.M., when UVR intensity is greatest. (Actually, wide time zones, seasonal changes, and daylight savings time make your watch an unreliable guide to the sun's intensity. A more reliable indicator is the length of your shadow. The period of greatest sun intensity is when the sun is halfway between the horizon and its zenith. During this period, shadows on level surfaces are shorter than the objects that cast them. The shorter the shadow, the more directly overhead the sun is, and the more intense its rays are. Use this rule of thumb: Stay out of the sun, or at least cover up and apply sunscreen, when your shadow is shorter than you are tall.) Fish and water-ski in the early morning and late afternoon. And, since 80 percent of UVR penetrates a foot of water, you'd be wise to schedule your snorkeling and scuba-diving activities for these hours, too. If your boat has a Bimini cover, put it up and stay under it.

2. When you do go out in the sun, wear *protective clothing*: a visored hat, tight-weave, dyed, long-sleeve shirts, and long pants. Dry, tight-weave clothing blocks virtually all UVR, but wet white clothing transmits nearly all UVR.

3. *Use sunscreens.* They bind with proteins in the outer layer of your skin to form an invisible barrier to UVR. An SPF 15 sunscreen containing PABA and a benzophenone (oxybenzone) can prevent sunburn, prevent premature aging, and cut your risk of skin cancer dramatically. Here are some tips on how to use sunscreens.

a. Use a sunscreen with an SPF (sun protection factor) of 15 or higher. The SPF number indicates the relative protection conferred by the sunscreen compared to bare skin, as determined under ideal laboratory conditions. (CAUTION! In actual use the SPF is probably only 50 to 75 percent of that specified on the label.)

b. Apply an ounce of the sunscreen to all exposed skin 20 minutes before you go out in the sun, using this formula: face and neck, ½ teaspoon; arms and shoulders, ½ teaspoon each side; torso, ½ teaspoon to front and back; legs and tops of feet, 1 teaspoon each side.

c. Use "waterproof" sunscreen when swimming or sweating, and reapply it every 80 minutes. (Wet skin burns more easily because water on the skin's surface reduces reflection of light.) Reapply "water resistant" sunscreens every 60 minutes.

d. Use sunscreen on cloudy, overcast days as well as on bright, sunny days.

e. Oral sunscreens are now available for individuals who are extremely photosensitive. These include beta-carotene (Solatene), chloroquine (Aralene), and some psoralen derivatives.

4. *Physical sunblocks* are opaque creams or pastes containing talc or zinc or titanium oxide. They block all solar radiation, but are too messy to apply to large areas. Just dab a little on the areas most likely to burn: nose, ears, cheeks, lips, thin areas of the scalp, and neck.

SUNBURN REMEDIES

The pain and itching of a severe sunburn will subside after a couple of days, but 48 hours can seem like an eternity when you are in agony. Here are some tried-and-true sunburn remedies.

1. A *cold shower* offers instant relief, but you probably don't have enough water on board to stay in the stall for 2 days.

2. *Cold compresses,* using a 50:50 solution of milk and ice water or Burow's solution, are soothing and anesthetic.

3. *Lotions,* such as Noxema, or Cetaphil with 0.25% menthol, help take away the sting and rehydrate the damaged epidermis.

4. *Analgesics,* such as aspirin, ibuprofen, and acetaminophen, take the edge off the pain. Severe burns may require a narcotic analgesic, such as Tylenol No. 3 or Vicodin. (Sunburn appears to be mediated by a group of chemicals called "prostaglandins," so either aspirin or ibuprofen—both prostaglandin inhibitors—theoretically should be more effective than acetaminophen.)

5. An *antihistamine,* such as diphenhydramine, 25 to 50 mg every 6 hours, will quell the itching associated with sunburn.

6. *Hydrocortisone cream,* 1% applied twice a day helps tame severe photosensitivity reactions.

7. *Prednisone,* 40 mg a day for 2 to 4 days, ameliorates the symptoms of "sun poisoning."

8. *Anesthetic sprays* offer short-term relief, but may contain benzocaine, which can be a photosensitizer. Using a medication with benzocaine would be like throwing gasoline on a fire.

•
•
•
•
•

14
DIVING MEDICINE

Loveliness unfathomable as ever lover saw in his young
bride's eye! Tell me not of thy teeth-tiered sharks, and thy
kidnapping ways. Let faith oust fact; let fancy oust memory;
I look deep down and do believe. [Starbuck, looking into the
Southern Ocean]

—Herman Melville, *Moby Dick*

Diving is a natural human pursuit. After all, we spend the first
nine months of our lives suspended in a miniature salt ocean, our
bodies are 57 percent salt water by weight, and as embryos we
recapitulate our evolution from sea dwellers to land animals by
briefly sporting gill slits and primordial tails.

But since our ancestors and fish went their separate evolutionary
ways, we have adapted to life on land. We long ago lost our
natural ability to cope with the coldness, darkness, wetness, air-
lessness, and hydrostatic pressure of the submarine world. But
while we have shed fins, gills, and air bladders, we have used our
formidable intelligence to open the door to Poseidon's kingdom.
To safely explore that kingdom, the diver must have a practical
understanding of the physical forces acting on his submerged body
and his body's physiologic response to those forces.

DIVING PHYSICS 101

At sea level, the weight of the air column extending from the
ground to the edge of space exerts a uniform pressure on our bodies
of 1 *atmosphere* (atm), or 14.7 pounds per square inch (psi). A 33-
foot column of sea water (FSW), or 34 feet of fresh water, exerts
the same pressure. If you dive to 99 feet in the Sea of Cortez, or
102 feet in Lake George, the total barometric pressure will be 4
atmospheres absolute (ATA, gauge plus atmospheric pressure).

If you ascend 33 feet, or 3,330 feet, in a balloon, you won't be aware of any change in the ambient pressure. When you dive underwater, you notice the increasing ambient pressure long before you reach a depth of 33 feet, where the ambient pressure is 2 atm.

Your tissues are comprised mostly of water, which is nearly incompressible, so they are immune to direct pressure effects. However, the gases dissolved in your blood and the air-filled spaces of the body, including your ears, nose, sinuses, lungs, and gastrointestinal tract, are directly affected by changes in ambient pressure. You can use the gas laws to predict the behavior of these gases.

Boyle's Law

At a constant temperature, the volume of a gas is inversely proportional to its pressure. This is represented by the equation

$$PV = K$$

where P = pressure, V = volume, and K is a constant.

Doubling the pressure of a gas halves its volume. Conversely, its volume doubles when you reduce its pressure by half. As you can see from Figure 23 on the following page, these pressure/ volume changes are most significant near the surface.

Dalton's Law

The pressure of a mixture of gases is the sum of the partial pressures of the components of the mixture. The pressure exerted by each gas is the same as it would be if that gas alone occupied the same volume. For air, which is 79 percent nitrogen (N) and 21 percent oxygen (O_2), Dalton's law can be expressed as

$$P(t) = P(O_2) + P(N_2) + P(x)$$

where $P(t)$ is the total ambient pressure, $P(O_2)$ is the partial pressure of oxygen, $P(N_2)$ is the partial pressure of nitrogen, and $P(x)$ is the partial pressure of the remaining gases in the air mixture. Dalton's law helps explain *decompression sickness*. The amount of

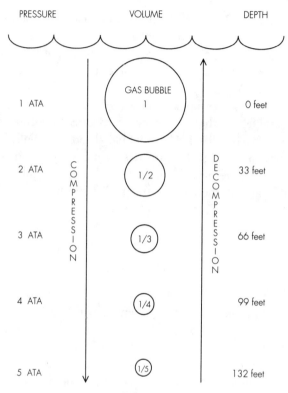

FIGURE 23
Boyle's Law—The volume of a gas is inversely proportional to its pressure at a given temperature.

ATA = atmosphere absolute
The diver's pressure gauge will read "1 atm" pressure at 33 feet, for example. But, the absolute pressure is 2 ATA (pressure of atmosphere plus pressure of 33 feet of water).

gas dissolved in a liquid depends on its partial pressure, which fluctuates with changes in ambient pressure.

Henry's Law

At a constant temperature, the amount of gas dissolved in a liquid is proportional to the pressure of the gas with which it is in equilibrium. That is,

$$\% Y = [P(Y)/P(t)] \times 100$$

where % Y is the amount of gas Y dissolved in a given volume of liquid, P(Y) is the partial pressure of Y, and P(t) is the total ambient pressure. You see Henry's law in action every time you open a bottle of soda. When you open the cap, the gas pressure in the neck of the bottle plummets and the gas dissolved in the soda returns to the gaseous state. Likewise, as you descend in water, ambient pressure increases and nitrogen in the compressed air you breathe dissolves in your blood and tissues. If you ascend too rapidly, the partial pressure of nitrogen decreases precipitously and nitrogen dissolved in the body bubbles out of solution.

DIVING SYNDROMES

Sharks, hypothermia, and falling anchors aren't the only things a diver needs to worry about. He also has to be wary of *dysbarism*. This is a group of pressure-related disorders that can turn diving into a nightmare.

Breath-hold Blackout

A sturdy and experienced swimmer volunteered to examine a mooring anchor on the sea bed at a depth of 50 feet. He took twelve deep breaths to reduce his alveolar carbon dioxide and dived in. He remembers swimming down and looking at the anchor but passed out as he turned to come up. A companion with a breathing set, seeing he had not surfaced in four minutes, swam down and found him lying prone and unconscious. He was brought to the surface very cyanosed and was revived with artificial ventilation.

—Dr. Stanley Miles, *Safety and Survival at Sea*

Breath-hold blackout is shallow water blackout (see Chapter 8) aggravated by pressure effects on gases within the lungs. Here's what happened to this breath-hold diver: He hyperventilated before his dive in order to lower his blood carbon dioxide level and thus blunt his urge to breathe. Then, strenuous swimming while underwater caused his blood oxygen level to *fall* rapidly, while his carbon dioxide level slowly rose. As he started to ascend, the ambient pressure decreased, as did the partial pressures of the oxygen and carbon dioxide in his lungs. Following the dictates of Henry's law, the decreased partial pressures of oxygen and carbon dioxide in his lungs caused a further lowering of the blood levels of these two gases, and the diver passed out because of lack of oxygen. He could have avoided all the fuss by taking just one or two—instead of twelve—deep breaths before diving.

BAROTRAUMA

Barotrauma is a group of related injuries sustained when a diver fails to or cannot maintain pressure equilibrium in the air-containing spaces of his body during a dive. It's the most common disorder of divers and can develop during descent or ascent.

Barotrauma of Descent

As you descend in water, the pressure on your body increases. The pressure in the air-containing spaces remains in balance with ambient pressure *if* they are vented. If these spaces are *not* vented, and they can't collapse, they are "squeezed" by the unopposed water pressure. Here are the squeeze syndromes you might experience on descent.

Mask Squeeze
You need to exhale from your nose every once in a while during a descent in order to keep the pressure inside your mask equal to ambient pressure. If you don't, capillaries in the skin and sclerae (whites of the eyes) will rupture, causing skin hemorrhages and bloodshot eyes.

Ear-Canal Squeeze
If wax, ear plugs, or a tight hood prevent water from entering your ear canals during a dive, the air in the canal will be compressed (Boyle's law), and pressure in the middle ear will cause the eardrum to bulge outward. You'll get an earache, blood blisters in the ear canal, and bleeding or rupture of the ear drum.

Treatment

Give Cortisporin otic suspension, 3 to 4 drops in each ear four times a day, if the injury occurred in polluted water, and analgesics. Put a moratorium on diving until the symptoms resolve.

Prevention

Don't allow wax to build up in your ears, break the seal on your diving hood to allow water to enter the external canal before diving, and don't use ear plugs.

Middle-Ear Squeeze

If you "equalize" by swallowing or by performing a "Valsalva maneuver" (exhaling against closed lips and nostrils) every few feet during descent, you will force air through the eustachian tubes and into the middle ears, and the pressure in the ears will remain in equilibrium with environmental pressure. If you forget to equalize, or your eustachian tubes are blocked because of a cold or allergies, a relative vacuum develops in the middle ear and the eardrum will bulge inward (see Figure 24). You'll get a "full"

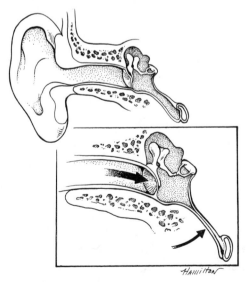

FIGURE 24
Middle-ear squeeze.

feeling in the ears, loss of hearing, bleeding from the ears, and wicked pain as the eardrum stretches and bulges inward. The pain will disappear if you ascend a few feet and equalize. If you continue to descend, the drum may rupture, and that can spell disaster. Cold water in the middle ear can cause severe vertigo, vomiting, disorientation, panic, and drowning.

Treatment
Pseudoephedrine, 60 mg every 6 hours for 5 days will reduce the congestion in the middle ear, and antihistamines or a nasal spray (Afrin, 2 sprays twice a day) will help control allergies. If the eardrum ruptures, take amoxicillin, 250 mg every 8 hours for 10 days. And don't resume diving until all symptoms have abated. Diving with an incompletely healed eardrum perforation can be deadly.

Prevention
Ventilate the middle ear by performing a Valsalva maneuver or the Frenzel maneuver (swallowing with a closed glottis, mouth and nostrils) every few feet while descending.

Inner-Ear Barotrauma
If you are overly exuberant in your attempts to equalize, you may rupture the round or oval window of the inner ear and develop sudden hearing loss, vertigo, and ringing in the ear.

Treatment
This is a serious disorder and must be treated by an ear, nose, and throat specialist ASAP. In the meantime, keep the victim at bed rest with his head elevated, and tell him not to strain.

Sinus Squeeze
The paranasal sinuses communicate with the respiratory passages through little openings called "ostia." Normally, the ostia remain open and the sinuses equalize automatically during a dive. But if the sinuses are congested, and you can't equalize during descent, a relative vacuum develops in the sinuses that can cause severe

pain and bleeding from the nose. *Treatment* and *prevention* are the same as for middle-ear squeeze.

Barotrauma of Ascent

As you *ascend,* Boyle's law dictates that the air in your sinuses, ears, intestines, and lungs expands as the ambient pressure decreases. If air isn't vented from these spaces, the expanding air can cause a number of problems.

If you can equalize well enough during descent to avoid middle-ear squeeze, you shouldn't have any ear problems on ascent, *unless* you have a cold and the medication you took prior to diving wears off before you ascend. In that case, you may suffer from "reverse middle-ear squeeze." Treatment is the same as for middle-ear squeeze.

If unequal middle-ear pressures develop during ascent, you may get *alternobaric vertigo* (ABV). ABV resolves as soon as you equalize your middle ears (try pinching your nostrils and swallowing).

Air trapped under a filling during descent may expand during ascent and cause *tooth squeeze.* The pain will suddenly disappear if the tooth explodes. Conversely, the tooth might *implode* during descent if a pocket of air under a filling doesn't equilibrate with ambient pressure.

If your pre-dive meal consisted of beans or carbonated beverages, you might be the victim of *gastrointestinal barotrauma* ("gas in the gut") as gas in the intestines expands during ascent. You'll have abdominal fullness, belching, flatulence, and, possibly, cramping abdominal pain. "Gas in the gut" can lead to shock and loss of consciousness, but these symptoms are unlikely if you vent excess bowel gas during your ascent.

"Burst Lung": The Pulmonary Overpressurization Syndrome (POPS)

If you hold your breath as you ascend, expanding air in your lungs will stretch and tear the lung tissues and air will escape from the *alveoli,* the terminal air sacs of the lungs. The worst possible time to hold your breath during an ascent is when you are within a few feet of the surface. Air in your lungs expands far out of proportion to the change in depth near the surface, and you can get "burst lung" while ascending from a depth of 4 feet if you hold your breath. POPS can take these forms.

1. *Mediastinal Emphysema.* Emphysema is swelling or inflation due to the presence of air. Air from ruptured alveoli may travel to the *mediastinum* (the root of the lung) and to the base of the neck, causing hoarseness, chest pain, coughing up of blood, fullness in the neck, shortness of breath, difficulty swallowing, and *subcutaneous emphysema* (air under the skin). Rarely, air moves into the pleural space between the chest wall and lung, causing a *pneumothorax* (see Chapter 4). *Treatment* for mediastinal emphysema consists of bed rest.

2. *Dysbaric Air Embolism (DAE).* An air embolism is an air bubble in the blood; it can disable or kill a diver. Air bubbles from ruptured alveoli enter the pulmonary veins and then pass through the heart and into the arterial circulation. These air emboli can lodge in small blood vessels anywhere in the body and obstruct circulation beyond that point. They usually float "upstream" into the brain, because the diver's head is upright, but they can also lodge in the coronary arteries and precipitate a heart attack. DAE classically afflicts a diver who runs out of air and ascends quickly to the surface while holding his breath, or a novice diver who panics at the sight of a shark and blasts to the surface like a Poseidon missile.

DAE strikes suddenly and dramatically after surfacing. The diver may break the surface of the water, gasp, lose consciousness, and sink back under the waves. He may have a seizure or appear to be having a stroke. Paralysis, headache, confusion, blindness, and loss of sensation are common symptoms.

Treatment
First, have the victim lie on his left side with his head down to prevent bubbles from entering his heart or brain. Then arrange for evacuation to a hyperbaric chamber for recompression PDQ (pretty darn quick). *NOTE:* Call the National Diver's Alert Network (DAN) at Duke University (1-919-684-8111) for advice.

Prevention
Breathe normally throughout your ascent, and ascend slowly for the last 10 feet. If you run out of air, exhale continuously as you ascend.

DECOMPRESSION SICKNESS (DCS)

DCS, a.k.a. "the bends," is caused by nitrogen bubbles forming in the blood and body tissues during ascent. These bubbles can pop up in blood vessels or tissues anywhere in the body and make you feel as though you've been embraced by the Iron Maiden of Nuremburg.

As you descend underwater, rising ambient pressure increases the partial pressure of nitrogen in the alveoli. This increased gas pressure creates a gradient as it drives nitrogen into solution in your blood and tissues, in compliance with Henry's law:

N in alveoli → blood → tissues

The longer and deeper you dive, the more nitrogen dissolves in your tissues. During a controlled ascent, a gradient is established whereby nitrogen dissolved in the tissues moves first into the blood, and then into the lungs, where it is exhaled as a gas:

N in tissues → blood → alveoli → gas

During a hasty ascent, a precipitous drop in ambient pressure causes the tissues to become *supersaturated* with nitrogen; that is, the gas pressure within the tissues is suddenly greater than the pressure surrounding the dissolved nitrogen. Bubbles form in the blood and tissues, just as a bottle of ginger ale turns bubbly when you remove the cap:

N dissolved in tissues + blood → N gas bubbles

These nitrogen bubbles obstruct blood vessels wherever they form and also trigger an intense inflammatory reaction which leads to the *sludging* (thickening) of blood in the capillaries and to tissue oxygen deprivation. Tissues supplied by these blood vessels are then deprived of oxygen and vital nutrients, and they die if the bubbles aren't forced back into solution by recompression.

Predisposing Factors for DCS

Diving in cold water, advanced age, poor physical condition, obesity, vigorous physical exercise underwater, cold water, multiple dives, trauma, and dehydration all increase your risk of DCS.

Symptoms

DCS symptoms may appear immediately after surfacing, but there is usually a delay of several minutes to several hours as nitrogen bubbles grow and tissue swelling increases. Since bubbles can form in any tissue, there may be a wide range of symptoms, but the central nervous and musculoskeletal systems take the big hits.

• *Limbs.* Joint pain ("joint bends") is the most common symptom of DCS. The shoulders and elbows are affected most often. The pain may be mild (the "niggles") or severe, may be made worse by movement of the joint, and is relieved by pressure. The joint appears normal.

• *Skin.* Mottling and marbling are harbingers of serious DCS.

• *Lungs.* Large numbers of bubbles in the pulmonary veins can obstruct the flow of oxygenated blood back to the heart and lead to the "chokes." Symptoms include burning substernal chest pain, cough, and shortness of breath. The chokes are rare, but may be fatal if the victim isn't recompressed in a hyperbaric chamber ASAP.

• *Central nervous system.* Bubbles can form anywhere within the brain and spinal cord and cause *any* neurologic symptom. Spinal-cord injuries are common in DCS victims and may start as back pain radiating to the abdomen shortly after surfacing. Then you get a "pins and needles" feeling in your legs, have trouble emptying your bladder, and feel unsteady on your feet. Finally, you become paralyzed from the waist down. The paralysis can be reversed if you are treated promptly in a hyperbaric chamber. DCS can also cause blurred or double vision, tunnel vision, partial blindness, migraine-like headaches, inappropriate behavior, and the "staggers" (vertigo).

Treatment

Any diver with DCS, even if his symptoms are mild, needs to be transported to a hyperbaric chamber as quickly as possible. Have someone get on the radio to summon help from the Coast Guard while you tend to the victim. If you have oxygen and IV equipment on board, give him 100% oxygen. Then start an infusion of Ringer's lactate or 0.9% normal saline. If you can, insert a Foley catheter and infuse the IV fluids at a rate sufficient to maintain urine output at 1 to 2 mL/kg/hour. If you can't start an IV, encourage the victim to drink plenty of fluids. Keep him warm, give him 5 grains of aspirin to help break up clots in the capillaries, and analgesics as needed.

Prevention

Treating decompression sickness is like trying to get toothpaste back into the tube. Even if you get to a hyperbaric chamber quickly, recompression is not always completely effective. Healing may require weeks or months, and you may be left with a permanent disability that will disqualify you from further diving. Better an ounce of prevention than a few atmospheres of cure. Here are some ways to avoid DCS.

1. Use the U.S. Navy decompression tables. Pad the tables by using the next greater depth, regardless of how much time was spent at shallower depths. (That is, use the next greater depth in the tables to figure your decompression time.) When diving at altitude, use special decompression tables that require longer decompression times.

2. Never ascend faster than 1 foot per second, and make a 3-minute or longer safety stop at 10 FSW at the conclusion of repetitive dives, or on any dive over 60 FSW.

3. On repetitive dives, descend to shallower depths with each succeeding dive, and "jump tables" so that you spend less time at any given depth than on previous dives.

4. Stay well-hydrated on the days that you dive to keep dissolved nitrogen flowing through your capillaries. Dark, scanty urine indicates dehydration; clear urine is a sign of adequate hydration.

5. Refrain from heavy work or exercise for at least 6 hours after diving.

6. Don't fly for at least 12 hours after "no recompression" diving, or 24 hours if decompression stops were required during ascent.

NITROGEN NARCOSIS

Jacques Cousteau called it "rapture of the deep"; some divers call it "the narks." Call it whatever you like, as long as you understand that nitrogen narcosis is *dangerous*. Nitrogen is an inert gas, but it has an anesthetic or narcotic effect when it's inhaled at high partial pressures. It has an intoxicating effect, not unlike alcohol. According to "Martini's law," each 50-foot increase in depth produces the same effect as one martini on an empty stomach. *Symptoms* start at 75 to 100 FSW with light-headedness, euphoria, and impairment of judgment. Mental functioning, reasoning ability, and manual dexterity nose-dive at greater depths. Your reaction time slows; you may lose your mouth piece and become disoriented between 200 to 300 feet. At greater depths, you will hallucinate and black out.

Treatment
Ascend to a depth above 100 FSW. Symptoms always resolve before you reach the surface.

•
•
•
•
•

15

INSOMNIA AND SLEEP DEPRIVATION

*When I came to . . . I realized that the sloop was plunging
into a heavy sea, and looking out of the companionway, to
my amazement saw a tall man at the helm. . . . One may
imagine my astonishment. His rig was that of a foreign sailor,
and the large red cap he wore was cockbilled over his left ear,
and all was set off with shaggy black whiskers. He would
have been taken for a pirate in any part of the world. While
I gazed upon his threatening aspect I forgot the storm, and
wondered if he had come to cut my throat. This he seemed
to divine. "Señor," said he, doffing his cap, "I have come
to do you no harm. . . . I am one of Columbus's crew.
. . . I am the pilot of the PINTA come to aid you. Lie
quiet, Señor captain," he added, "and I will guide your ship
to-night."*

—Joshua Slocum, *Sailing Alone Around the World*

Missing a night's sleep now and then never hurt anyone. However, chronic sleeplessness can lead to disaster. No one knows
how many solo trans-Atlantic sailors or circumnavigators have
perished at sea over the years because of fatal lapses in judgment
induced by chronic sleep deprivation.

SLEEP AND PERFORMANCE

The ancient Romans had a punishment known as "waking torture," which they used to execute King Perseus of Macedonia.
Insomnia torture was used in the Middle Ages to extract confes-
sions and drive out demons. During the Korean War, the Chinese
broke down the resistance of captured American pilots by keeping
them awake for long periods. Losing one night's sleep may make

you crabby, but it won't significantly affect your ability to plot a course or take a bearing. Several nights of poor sleep, however, will slow your thinking, impair your judgment and memory, and dull your reflexes, making many routine shipboard chores hazardous. Chronic insomnia can take the fun out of long cruises and ruin your health.

SLEEP PHYSIOLOGY 101

Sleep should be measured in terms of quality, not quantity. Forget that old saw about everyone needing eight hours of sleep a night. A good night's sleep will leave you feeling restored and refreshed in the morning, regardless of how many hours you spent in the bunk. Napoleon, Thomas Edison, and Winston Churchill got a lot done on three or four hours sleep a night, while Albert Einstein needed ten to keep the creative wheels turning. You have to find out for yourself how many hours you need.

The early Germanic tribes believed that sleep and death were brothers. In the computer age, it's easier to think of sleep as the daily period when the brain catches up on its data processing. Sleep researchers studying brain wave recordings have learned that there are two stages of sleep, nonrapid eye movement (NREM) and rapid eye movement sleep (REM), which alternate in 90-minute cycles throughout the night. The first stages of sleep are NREM sleep, which is deep sleep. It seems to play a role in body recovery. REM sleep, which is light sleep, follows NREM sleep. You dream during REM sleep, and as you do, your eyes move about rapidly. REM sleep seems to be important for mental recovery. When it's disrupted, you become anxious and irritable. Alcohol and sleeping pills interfere with normal REM sleep.

Sleep Rhythms

Sleep is one of many bodily functions that has a daily, or "circadian" rhythm (from Latin *circa dies*, "about a day"). You have an internal body clock that governs everything from body temperature to blood hormone levels to cellular metabolism. Problems arise when this clock does not keep perfect time. Some people's body clocks tend to run a little slow, others' run a little fast. People who have slow clocks are called "owls." Owls have a hard time falling asleep before three or four in the morning, but sleep normally once they nod off. They function fairly well when they are on a regular sleep-wake cycle, but get into trouble when they go on a cruise. Standing four-hour watches at all times of the day and night does violence to their circadian rhythms. After a few days at sea, their body clocks are totally desynchronized. They rarely go to bed at the same time two days in a row and may never get a chance to sleep for more than four hours in a row. "Larks," on the other hand, have fast body clocks. They turn in early and rise at the crack of dawn. They have fewer problems adjusting to the irregular sleep hours dictated by the demands of sailing a boat and adapt better to watch routine.

Shipboard watch routine isn't the only way to screw up your circadian rhythms. Sleeping in on the weekends and during vacations will do it too. Your circadian rhythms adapt to a longer sleep cycle, and then have to make a sudden switch back to a shorter cycle on Monday morning or at the end of the vacation.

Jet Lag

Overseas travel can also throw a monkey wrench into your normal sleep rhythm. If you fly from New York to Helsinki, Finland, to take delivery on a new ocean racer, you'll travel across seven time zones. Your biological clock will be out of synch with local time. You'll be ready to turn in about the time you reach the boat yard, and you'll feel crabby and sluggish until you reset your body clock. This is what is meant by *jet lag*. If you fly down to Argentina to spend a few days cruising the Gulf of San Matias, on the other hand, you'll travel 6,000 miles, but cross only two time zones. Jet lag won't be as much of a problem.

The best way to reset your body clock after transoceanic or transcontinental travel is to immediately switch to the new time.

If you spend most of your time outdoors soaking up sunlight, your body clock will advance to local time within three days. (Light is what sleep researchers call a *zeitgeber*, or "timegiver," a powerful signal that resets the body clock.)

Aggravating Factors

Insomia can also be caused by the following.

1. *Psychological problems.* If you often wake up early in the morning and have difficulty falling back to sleep, have poor self-esteem, feel melancholy, and have lost interest in friends, food, and sex, you are probably depressed. If you feel tense and nervous, worry excessively, and have trouble falling asleep at night, you may be suffering from chronic anxiety, which can be a symptom of depression. You should seek professional help if you think you are suffering from either anxiety or depression.

2. *Medical problems.* Asthma, arthritis, headache, hay fever, low-back pain, and seasickness can all keep you awake at night. So can kidney problems, thyroid disorders, anemia, diabetes, reflux esophagitis, peptic ulcer, carbon monoxide poisoning, and any acute, painful injury. Medications that can interfere with the normal sleep cycle include antihistamines, diet pills, certain antidepressants, asthma medications, thyroid medications, steroid preparations, some blood pressure medications, medications containing caffeine, DOPA, and sleeping pills, and sedatives (you may experience a "rebound insomnia" when you stop taking them).

3. *Lifestyle factors.* These factors include the following.

a. Caffeine. There's nothing like a steaming mug of black coffee to get your motor running when you go on watch at midnight. But your motor may not slow down at 4 A.M. when you're ready to turn in. And caffeine sensitivity increases with age. Many soft drinks and medications (including analgesics, cold preparations, and diet pills) contain caffeine.

b. Tobacco. Nicotine is a powerful stimulant, and many smokers are insomniacs.

c. Alcohol. A nightcap may make you sleepy, but alcohol fragments your sleep, causing frequent awakenings during the night.

d. Stress. A harried, tension-filled life-style is incompatible with normal sleep. It's normal to feel stressed out while fighting your way westward through the Strait of Magellan. But you may need to rearrange your life or talk to your doctor about stress management and relaxation techniques if you feel that life is a continuous maelstrom.

4. *Poor sleep habits.* Joseph Stalin had several different bedrooms and would move from one to another during the night to elude would-be assassins. It's hard to get into the proper frame of mind for sleep when you think you might be shot during the night. Here are some good sleep habits you should try to develop.

a. Sleep in the same bunk every night. Your cabin should be quiet, dark, and adequately heated. Your mattress should be firm, and your sheets and pillow comfortable. And don't forget to rig your lee cloth.

b. Don't go to bed until you are sleepy. Get up when you are done sleeping.

c. Relax for an hour or so before going to bed.

d. Don't *try* to sleep. You cannot will yourself to sleep. It's better to get up and look at the stars, listen to soothing music, or read a book than to toss and turn all night.

e. Avoid big meals before bedtime.

f. Don't drink or smoke within 3 or 4 hours of bedtime.

g. Cut down on your caffeine consumption, and don't drink coffee or tea within 6 hours of bedtime.

h. Consult with your doctor if you think a medical problem is interfering with your sleep.

i. Drink a glass of milk at bedtime (calcium is a natural sedative).

j. Thirty minutes of vigorous physical exercise each day is the best prescription for insomnia. You fall asleep quicker and sleep more soundly when you are physically tired. And exercise triggers the release of *endorphins*, natural mood elevators that give you a sense of well-being and banish depression. Exercise in late afternoon or early evening for best effect. Swimming, calisthenics, jumping rope, and jogging or walking (when ashore) are all excellent exercise. And a good massage just before bedtime will help you to relax.

k. Both Winston Churchill and John Kennedy had a talent for taking catnaps anytime they wished. Try to develop a facility for taking frequent short naps when at sea, particularly when thick weather is in the offing.

l. If you are planning a solo voyage, install a durable and dependable self-steering mechanism.

m. Try counting sheep—or dolphins.

Sleeping Pills (Hypnotics)

There are a number of over-the-counter and prescription medications that will help you to get to sleep. However, the agent that will send you gently off into the arms of Morpheus, keep you asleep all night, and not interfere with your normal sleep cycle has yet to be invented. Antihistamines, such as Dramamine and Benadryl, and long-acting prescription hypnotics and sedatives, such as Valium, Librium, and Dalmane, will make you sleepy, but you will wake up feeling hung over and more tired than when you went to bed.

Triazolam (Halcion) is an effective and safe hypnotic if used appropriately. It helps you to fall asleep, reduces nocturnal awakenings, and increases the duration of sleep. And it's metabolized quickly, so the hangover effect is minimal. It has a shorter half-life than alprazolam (Xanax), a popular sedative, and may even help you to remain alert the following day. However, it can cause early morning awakening and daytime anxiety. The dosage is 0.125 to 0.25 mg at bedtime. (*WARNING!* Rebound insomnia and withdrawal symptoms can occur after abrupt discontinuance of triazolam. To avoid these complications, use it intermittently rather than every night.)

·
·
·
·
·

16

FISH POISONING

"Here's a pretty kettle of fish!"

—Sir William S. Gilbert, *Iolanthe*

Chauncey Gotrocks was on a fishing vacation in the Bahamas. His mate had taken him out to a shallow reef that morning in the launch, and he had used a wet fly to catch a burly barracuda. He handed the fish over to his chef that afternoon when he returned to his yacht and feasted on Cajun-style baked barracuda that evening. Anticipating another day of great fishing, Chauncey turned in early that night. He awoke three hours later bathed in sweat and with an ominous rumbling in his belly. The rumbling turned into gut-wrenching cramps, vomiting, and explosive diarrhea. Then he got an odd tingling sensation in his lips, tongue, and throat. And his arms and legs felt strangely cold, even though he was sweating. His stomach settled down after a few hours, and he staggered back to the galley the next morning and described his symptoms to the chef. The chef told him it wasn't uncommon in the Caribbean for people to become ill after eating large reef fish such as barracuda, red snapper, and grouper. They called it "ciguatera poisoning."

The sea is a vast treasure trove of culinary delights. But if you're going to dine at Neptune's table, beware: There are some nasty surprises hidden among all those tasty offerings. Ciguatera, scombroid, and other kinds of fish poisoning can cause gastrointestinal horrors for the nautical gastronome. Here's a look at some of these piscatorial poisoners.

CIGUATERA POISONING

Ordinarily, it's better to be at the end of the food chain, but I'd rather be at the end of an *anchor* chain than a food chain that begins with *Gambierdiscus toxicus.* This dinoflagellate produces *ciguatoxin* and *maitotoxin,* two poisons which accumulate in the flesh, blood, and viscera of larger fish higher up the food chain. If you're the final link in such a food chain, you will get violently sick.

CIGUATOXIC FISH

Amberjack	Parrotfish
Anchovy	Porgy
Barracuda	Sailfish
Croaker	Sea bass
Dolphin	Snapper
Flounder	Surgeonfish
Grouper	Swordfish
Herring	Tarpon
Inshore tuna	Triggerfish
Moray eel	Wrasse
Mullet	

Ciguatoxic fish are bottom-dwellers, reef fish that cruise the warm waters from 35 degrees north latitude to 35 degrees south latitude. There are over five hundred known ciguatoxic species (see table above) but it's the big bruisers (tarpon, groupers, amberjack, and barracuda) that you've really got to be wary of. Their meat and organs have the highest concentrations of ciguatoxin. But it's almost impossible to tell if any given fish contains the toxins. For one thing, fish of the same species caught in neighboring waters may be toxic in one area but not in the other. And the toxins themselves are colorless, odorless, and tasteless. And indestructible. You can fry, boil, steam, stew, or broil these fish— it doesn't matter. Nothing short of a nuclear device will deactivate ciguatoxin and maitotoxin.

Symptoms

Ciguatoxin causes prolonged stimulation of the nervous system. Fifteen minutes to three hours after eating ciguatoxic fish, you'll break out in a drenching sweat and develop gut-wrenching abdominal cramps, watery diarrhea, headache, and bizarre neurological symptoms. These include numbness and tingling in the lips, mouth, and throat; a sensation of "carbonation" during swallowing; a feeling of loose, painful teeth; temporary blindness; nightmares; hallucinations; muscle twitching; and a weird reversal of temperature sensation (the "dry ice phenomenon"). Ice and other cold objects will feel hot, and warm objects will feel cold. (One man reportedly felt compelled to blow onto an ice cream cone to cool it down so it wouldn't burn his tongue!) In severe poisonings, respiratory paralysis results in death. Itching, muscle aches, tingling in the arms and legs, and temperature reversal may persist for weeks, months, or years. Drinking alcoholic beverages, eating nontoxic fish, stress, and severe illness have been known to provoke a recurrence of itching and other symptoms years later. And the toxin accumulates in human flesh, so that you can expect to have an even more intense reaction the next time you dine on ciguatoxic fish.

Treatment
There's no magic bullet for ciguatera poisoning. Vomiting can be controlled with promethazine (one 25-mg suppository every 6 hours as needed), and the victim should be encouraged to drink fluids once his stomach has settled down. If he shows no signs of improving after several hours, he should be evacuated to a hospital. Don't let him drink alcohol or eat nuts, fish, or shellfish for 2 weeks after the poisoning. These can all cause a relapse.

Prevention
You won't get ciguatera poisoning if you don't eat predatory reef fish, especially the organs and roe, and especially those over 6 pounds. If you have an insatiable craving for these fish, first give a small portion to a cat or another small animal. If the animal vomits, fire up the grill and make hamburgers for dinner.

SCOMBROID POISONING (THE "MAHI-MAHI FLUSH")

The "mahi-mahi flush" is not a poker hand. It's a sobriquet for *scombroid* poisoning, the most common type of fish poisoning worldwide. The rogues' gallery of scombrotoxic fish includes members of the scombroideae family (tuna, swordfish, bonito, mackerel, skipjack, and albacore) as well as such nonscombroid fish as mahi-mahi (dolphin), herring, sardines, and bluefish (see table below). All of these fish have high concentrations of the amino acid histidine in their dark meat. Histidine itself is harmless, but if the fish is not properly refrigerated after being caught, surface bacteria break the amino acid down into histamine and saurine. These are heat-stable toxins that are not destroyed by cooking. Scombrotoxic fish usually look, smell, and taste perfectly normal, although they often will have a sharply metallic or peppery flavor.

SCOMBROTOXIC FISH

Scombroid Fish	Nonscombroid Fish
Bonito	Amberjack
Kingfish	Anchovy
Mackerel	Black marlin
Needlefish	Bluefish
Saury	Herring
Swordfish	Kahawai
Tuna (albacore,	Mahi-mahi (dolphin)
bluefin, and yellowfin)	Pilchard
Wahoo	Sardine

The histamine in spoiled dark-meat fish causes a histamine reaction. Histamine is a powerful chemical that mediates allergic reactions. It causes capillaries in the skin and mucous membranes to dilate and leak fluids into the tissues and stimulates intense itching in these tissues. In a *true* allergic reaction, an external stimulus (such as pollen or bee venom) stimulates the body to release endogenous histamine. In scombroid poisoning, the histamine comes from an exogenous source but causes a reaction that is indistinguishable from a true allergic reaction, and so it is called a "pseudoallergic reaction."

Symptoms

The unlucky person who unwittingly eats scombrotoxic fish has the Devil to pay and no pitch hot. Fifteen to 90 minutes after eating tainted fish, he'll develop deep-red flushing of his head, neck, and upper torso; itching; hives; red eyes; swelling of the face and throat; wheezing; nausea; vomiting; abdominal cramps; explosive diarrhea; headache; burning of the gums and throat; dizziness; palpitations; and faintness. The symptoms usually resolve within 8 to 12 hours, even without treatment. However, some people continue to have a lingering headache, abdominal cramps, diarrhea, insomnia, weakness, and loss of appetite for up to ten days.

Treatment

The best way to treat a histamine reaction is with an antihistamine. If the victim isn't vomiting, give him diphenhydramine (Benadryl), 50 mg by mouth, and repeat every 6 hours until his symptoms subside. If he *is* vomiting, give him a 25-mg promethazine suppository, wait until he stops vomiting, and then give him the diphenhydramine. If he becomes faint and pale and his pulse becomes weak, he has become hypotensive because of the action of the histamine and the loss of fluid from vomiting and diarrhea. Position him on the deck or in a bunk with his head down and feet elevated above heart level, and offer him fluids. If you happen to have some cimetidine (Tagamet) tablets on board, give him 300 mg every 6 hours until he feels well. Cimetidine is an antihistamine used to treat peptic ulcers, as are famotidine (Pepcid) and ranitidine (Zantac); any of these drugs will help neutralize the histamine reaction.

Prevention

Avoid scombroid poisoning by immediately gutting and cooling your catch. Toxic levels of scombrotoxins form within 3 or 4 hours at room temperature, so keep the fish on ice until it's ready for the broiler. Don't eat any fish that has a peppery or metallic taste, or the smell of ammonia.

CLUPEOTOXIN POISONING

Fish which feed on plankton (e.g., herring, sardines, bonefish, anchovies, ladyfish, and tarpon) sometimes contain *clupeotoxin*. This is an industrial-strength toxin. Dine on a clupeotoxic fish and you'll get a metallic taste in your mouth, then cotton mouth, violent vomiting and explosive diarrhea, abdominal cramps, headache, drenching sweats, seizures, and vise-like muscle cramps. Then you'll get dizzy, turn blue, go into shock, and, very possibly, die. This severe poisoning can be treated effectively only in a hospital. Avoid it by not eating clupeotoxic fish from Caribbean, coastal African, and Indo-Pacific waters during the summer months when toxicity is highest.

TETRODON POISONING

Many consider blowfish to be a gourmet food, especially in Japan, where it is served as "fugu." But eat it and you risk getting tetrodon poisoning. Blowfish, toadfish, balloonfish, and other pufferfish contain tetrodotoxin, an extremely potent poison that blocks nerve impulses and causes paralysis and death in 60 percent of cases. If you start to feel exhilarated and get a funny tingling feeling in your skin, tongue, and lips, excess salivation, headache, vomiting, and diarrhea after eating pufferfish, you'd better get yourself to the nearest hospital fast. Tetrodotoxin isn't destroyed by cooking, so you'd be smart to avoid eating pufferfish.

SHELLFISH POISONING

The bivalve mollusks (clams, mussels, oysters, and scallops) filter large volumes of water through their gills and siphons and extract oxygen and plankton. They also filter out viruses, bacteria, biological toxins, and chemical and radioactive waste, and concentrate them in their flesh and organs. Eating raw shellfish can cause:

• *Paralytic shellfish poisoning.* Dinoflagellates bloom during the "non-R" months (May through August) on the New England and West coasts and cause the infamous "red tides." These algae blooms kill birds and fish by the tons. Those shellfish that survive often harbor large quantities of *saxitoxin*, a potent neurotoxin, in their gills and digestive organs. Saxitoxin is virtually indestructible. You can't destroy it by cooking.

I'd rather be caught by a giant clam than get paralytic shellfish poisoning. Fifteen minutes to several hours after eating tainted shellfish, you get tingling of the lips, tongue, and gums that rapidly spreads to your neck, hands, and feet. Then you become dizzy, lightheaded, and nauseated, your teeth feel loose, and you have a devil of a time speaking and swallowing as paralysis sets in. You may become totally paralyzed and die of asphyxia, remaining awake and alert to the bitter end. Avoid going into a shell like that by eating shellfish only in months that end in the letter *R*.

• *Neurotoxic shellfish poisoning.* This milder form of paralytic shellfish poisoning is caused by the dinoflagellate *P. breve.* This one hits you up to three hours after the clambake and causes an illness similar to that caused by ciguatera poisoning. This poisoning can cause respiratory paralysis and needs to be treated in the hospital.

• *Gastroenteritis.* The Norwalk and other viruses cause abdominal cramps, vomiting, diarrhea, and fever 24 to 48 hours after the eating of contaminated shellfish. Vomiting can be controlled with promethazine suppositories, and diarrhea with Imodium tablets. The symptoms abate in a day or two. Depurating shellfish in sterile water is not a reliable way to purge them of viruses, unless you're willing to wait several weeks to eat them. And, while steaming clams at 100 degrees Celsius will destroy any virus or bacteria, be careful. The shells will open in 60 seconds, but the internal temperature of the clams will not reach 100 degrees until they've been steamed for 4 minutes.

17
VENOMOUS MARINE ANIMALS

Brendan maneuvered his skiff alongside the lobster buoy and shifted the engine into neutral. He leaned over the gunwale, hooked the line under the buoy with a gaff, and started pulling in the black polypropylene line. The water was ice cold, and the rope cut into his hands like a hacksaw. After a dozen hard pulls, the line became sluggish as the trap broke the surface of the water and lost some of its buoyancy. He reached down, grabbed the trap by the yoke, and swung it onto the deck. A quick glance told him there were no keepers; just a couple of "shorts" and a sundial. He threw the cover back in disgust and stuck his hand into the trap to evict the trespassers.

Suddenly, Brendan howled in pain and yanked his hand back as though he had touched a hot stove. He grabbed his wrist and looked at his hand in horror. Bright red blood spurted out of a vicious gash that ran from the second knuckle to his wrist. His face was transformed into a mask of pain. His hand swelled into an angry red pulp, and his nerve endings screamed in outrage. He looked into the trap to see what manner of beast had inflicted such a horrible wound. A stingray lay on the bottom of the trap, its fearsome 3-inch spine coated with Brendan's blood.

Brendan was painfully reminded that the fisherman casts his hook, net, or trap into a world whose denizens have a daunting array of cruel and ingenious ways to defend themselves. He risks being injured or killed by fish armed with spines, fangs, sharp snouts, and venomous fins and tentacles.

Brendan got a nasty surprise when he disturbed that stingray, but it could have been worse. Had he been fishing or swimming in the waters off Queensland, Australia, he might have had an encounter of the worst kind with the dreaded *box-jellyfish*, whose sting can kill a human in 30 seconds. If he had been casting his net in the Arabian Sea, he might have pulled in a swarming mass of *Enhydrina schistosa*, sea snakes whose venom is more deadly than that of the coral snake. Or, if he had been diving in Indo-Pacific waters, he might have had an encounter with the deadly stonefish, whose venom is as lethal as a cobra's. Let's don scuba gear and take a close up and personal look at some of these terrors of the deep.

STINGRAYS

While exploring Chesapeake Bay, Captain John Smith hopped out of a boat barefoot onto a stingray, which had the temerity to stick its dart into his leg. It was a foolish act on the part of the fish, for Smith was no common man. Instead of trying to get clear of it, Smith held it to the bottom with his foot, drew his hanger, hacked the fish to pieces and ate several collops raw.

—Horace Beck, *Folklore and the Sea*

Stingrays, the original demons of the deep, are the commonest cause of marine envenomations in the United States (nearly two thousand per year). Dubbed the "devilfish" by the ancients, stingrays are found in shallow coastal waters, particularly in sheltered bays, river mouths, and lagoons. They range in size from several inches to 12 feet and have flattened, diamond-shaped bodies with wing-like pectoral fins (see Figure 25). The business end of the stingray consists of one to four venomous stings, each 1 to 17 inches long, embedded in a long, whip-like tail. The sting has two rows of retrorse (backward-pointing) barbs and two grooves on its undersurface which contain venom glands. It's covered with a thick integumentary sheath which also contains venom glands, and whose surface may be coated with venom and mucus.

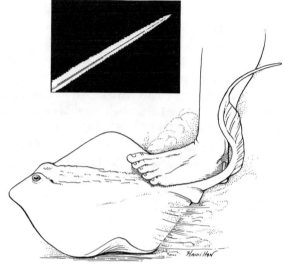

FIGURE 25
Stingray in action.

Sting Operation

Marine biologists insist that, despite its frightening appearance, the stingray is not an aggressive fish. That's like saying that a land mine is not an offensive weapon. When a stingray burrows into a sandy or muddy bottom in search of food, with only its eyes, breathing hole, and tail showing, it's virtually invisible. When an unsuspecting swimmer or fisherman steps on it, its tail reflexively snaps up and buries the spine in the victim's skin, causing a deep puncture wound or laceration. The integumentary sheath ruptures, and venom is released from the venom glands and driven deep into the wound, along with mucus and bacteria. The sheath and spine may be left in the wound as well.

Symptoms

Stingray injuries are no fun at all. Sharp, excruciating pain quickly spreads throughout the limb. It peaks an hour or so after the sting, and then slowly diminishes over a period of 6 to 48 hours. The barbed spine ravages the skin, and bleeding from the wound can be profuse. The injured area first turns dusky blue and then bright red. As the venom destroys fat and muscle, the wound swells. The venom dilates blood vessels throughout the body, causing the blood pressure to drop. This, together with the intense pain, may cause dizziness, fainting, weakness, nausea, and anxiety. Less common symptoms include vomiting, diarrhea, sweating, twitching of the muscles in the injured limb, pain in the groin or armpit, muscle cramps, headache, irregular heartbeat, and (rarely) paralysis, seizures, and death. Obviously, a swimmer who seizes or becomes paralyzed is in dire straits. Most stingray injuries involve the foot and ankle, but wounds to the chest, abdomen, and even the heart have been reported, and are often lethal.

Treatment

1. Irrigate the wound thoroughly with salt water. This washes out much of the mucus, bacteria, and venom, and helps to numb the wound.

2. Manually remove as much debris as possible, including the integumentary sheath and sting, if present.

3. Apply suction to the wound with a Sawyer Extractor. This may remove some of the venom.

4. Immerse the injured limb in hot water (110 to 115 degrees Fahrenheit, or as hot as the victim can stand) for 30 to 90 minutes, or until the pain is relieved. Heat inactivates the venom and relieves pain.

5. Re-examine the wound and remove any remaining debris.

6. These wounds tend to become infected, so they should generally be packed with sterile gauze and covered with a sterile dressing. You may elect to loosely close large lacerations with surgical staples.

7. Give the victim TMP-SMX, one tablet every 12 hours, or ciprofloxacin, 500 mg every 12 hours, for 2 days, to reduce the risk of wound infection.

8. Large, gaping wounds and injuries to tendons, blood vessels, or nerves require surgical repair.

Prevention

Only steel boots can protect you from the powerful lash of a stingray's tail. The best way to avoid stepping on one of these nautical booby traps is to shuffle your feet across the bottom when wading in shallow water. You'll raise enough sand to spook any lurking stingrays, and they'll take off before you can step on them.

SCORPION FISH

The name says it all. These bony fish are the most dangerous venomous fish in the sea. They secrete themselves in nooks and crannies on the sea bottom and blend, chameleon-like, into the background. Their dorsal, anal, and pelvic fins are tipped with eighteen venomous spines, similar in shape and structure to those of the stingray. When an unsuspecting swimmer or diver steps on or handles a scorpion fish, the spines puncture his skin and inject venom deep into his flesh. This extremely potent venom can paralyze voluntary, involuntary, and heart muscles.

Scorpion fish are abundant in the waters off the Florida Keys, southern California, and Hawaii, and in the Gulf of Mexico. There are three groups of scorpion fish. In order of increasing toxicity they are:

1. *Zebra fish* (lionfishes, turkey fishes, butterfly cods). These free-swimming denizens of coral reefs cause mild envenomation.

2. *Scorpion fish* (scorpion fish, sculpin, and bullpout; a.k.a. rockfishes, sea pigs, waspfishes, bullheads, blobs). These cleverly camouflaged fish lurk among rocks and seaweed on the bottom of shallow bays and coral reefs. Their stings cause moderately severe reactions.

3. *Stonefish* (alias devilfish, sea toads, goblin fishes, lump-fishes, lupos, and stingfishes). These guys float like a butterfly and sting like a cobra. They bury themselves under the sand or hide under rocks or amongst debris on the shallow bottoms of tidal pools or reefs in Indo-Pacific waters. You'd rather bump into a rabid porcupine than a stonefish. Its venom is cobralike, and it will attack if disturbed. Its stings cause severe, often lethal, envenomation.

Symptoms

Scorpion fish stings cause immediate, agonizing, pulsating, or burning pain that radiates centrally. The pain peaks in 60 to 90 minutes and diminishes over a period of 6 to 12 hours. (Stonefish stings are incredibly painful, causing the victim to writhe in agony, become delirious, and even pass out. And the pain may last for days.) The wound swells and turns blue with surrounding areas of redness and warmth. Over the ensuing days, blisters form and the area around the wound becomes numb. Regional lymph nodes may become tender and swollen within 15 minutes. The flesh often becomes infected and necrotic, and sloughs off after a few days. Other symptoms include nausea, vomiting, weakness, headache, sweating, loss of consciousness, restlessness, delirium, shortness of breath, tremors, convulsions, paralysis, heart failure, ventricular fibrillation, and death. The wound heals slowly over a period of months, often leaving an unsightly scar.

Treatment

Stonefish envenomations are treated exactly like stingray injuries. An antivenin is available for stonefish envenomations from the Commonwealth Serum Laboratories in Melbourne, Australia.

Prevention

It's hard to avoid accidental contact with an invisible fish, but try. Handle a dead scorpion fish as though it were a hand grenade; its venom remains potent for up to 48 hours. And stay a stone's throw from stonefish.

CATFISH

Catfish are a little different from most fish. They have no scales, are poor swimmers, and have whiskers. Among the thousand species of freshwater and saltwater catfish are the *astroblepin* of South America, which use suction-cup-like lips to climb cliffs, and the Amazonian *candiru*, which has a perturbing propensity for parasitizing the human urethra. Other catfish species are less talented, but many have venomous stingers in their dorsal and pectoral fin spines, including the freshwater Carolina mudtom, channel, white, blue, and brown bullhead. Saltwater stinging catfish include the oriental catfish, which pokes about in tall seaweed, and the common sea catfish, a bottom dweller.

Symptoms

Catfish stings pack a wallop. When the fish becomes excited, it locks its sharp spines in an erect position. When a fisherman handles the fish, a spine can penetrate the skin of the hand or forearm and inject venom into the wound. The pain, variously described as stinging, throbbing, or scalding, is agonizing. It lasts for 30 to 60 minutes, or up to 2 days in the case of multiple stings or a sting by a large, tropical catfish. The wound turns white, then blue, then red and swollen. Infection and gangrene can set in, as well as muscle spasm, nausea, vomiting, abdominal cramps, headache, and difficulty breathing. Severe stings can result in irregular heartbeat, convulsions, loss of consciousness, shortness of breath, and, rarely, death.

Treatment

Catfish stings are treated in the same way as stingray injuries. These fish hang out in slow-moving, muddy, bacteria-rich waters, so wound infections are common, including gangrene and osteomyelitis. Clean the wound thoroughly, remove all foreign matter, and pack it open. Start TMP-SMX, one tablet every 12 hours, at the first sign of infection (fever, increasing pain and redness around the wound, and pus). Deep puncture wounds and hand and foot wounds are at high risk for infection, so take the same dose of TMP-SMX for 2 days as prophylaxis.

Prevention
Always use a gaff to boat catfish, keep your hands away from the dorsal and pectoral fins, and watch where you walk. Catfish spines can penetrate shoes.

SPONGES

Sponges are animals, believe it or not. They don't bite, but they can give you a heck of a rash if you bump into them, an affliction called "sponge diver's disease." The Hawaiian or West Indian *fire sponge* is a yellow-vermilion-orange sponge found in the waters off Hawaii and the Florida Keys. The *red moss sponge* is native to northeastern U.S. waters.

Symptoms

Contact with these sponges can give you:

1. An itchy, poison-ivy-like rash, caused by a toxin released into the skin. The skin may blister, swell, and turn red. Joints in the area may also swell, and you may experience malaise, nausea, fever, chills, muscle cramps, and dizziness.

2. A burning rash caused by spicules of silica or calcium carbonate that have punctured the skin.

Treatment
1. Wash the affected area thoroughly with soap and water.
2. Remove the spicules with adhesive tape.
3. Apply dilute (5%) vinegar compresses for 30 minutes four times a day.
4. Cover the affected area with moisturizing cream or 1% hydrocortisone ointment.
5. Use diphenhydramine to control itching.

COELENTERATES

The coelenterates (hydroids, jellyfish, sea anemones, and corals) are spineless, radially symmetrical animals with special stinging cells *(nematocysts)* lining their tentacles or mouths (see Figure 26). These microscopic structures consist of a cyst filled with venomous fluid and a coiled thread. When triggered by either chemical or mechanical stimuli, the thread fires out of the cyst like a tiny harpoon and strikes with sufficient force (2 to 5 pounds per square inch) to penetrate skin and deposit a dollop of venom. Millions of nematocysts line the tentacles of jellyfish and Portuguese men-of-war, each a repository of venom that is a witch's brew of tissue-destroying and allergy-provoking enzymes.

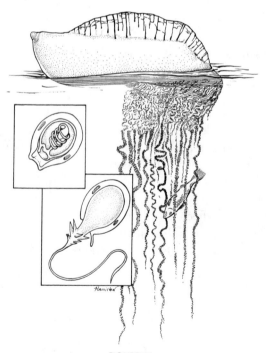

FIGURE 26
Portuguese man-of-war and nematocysts.

Hydroids

Contact with the *feather hydroid*, a plume-like animal, causes only mild skin irritation and itching.

A diver who steps on or handles *fire coral* (which is not a true coral) will suffer immediate burning pain, followed 30 minutes to several hours later by an itchy, red, bumpy rash or hives that slowly resolve over a period of days.

The *Portuguese man-of-war*, which drifts willy-nilly across warm, tropical waters throughout the Atlantic and Pacific oceans, is one of the more bizarre-looking life forms in the sea (see Figure 26). The only part of the animal you're likely to see is the iridescent purple sail, a 5- to 16-inch bladder filled with carbon monoxide and nitrogen monoxide which floats on the surface. Suspended from the sail are a number of long (up to 100 feet), clear, nematocyst-studded tentacles, which reach down into the depths, probing for prey. When an unsuspecting creature—fish or human—bumps into one of these nearly invisible tentacles, the impact triggers the release of hundreds of thousands of nematocysts.

Getting stung by a Portuguese man-of-war has been likened to being horse-whipped. The loving embrace of a man-of-war initially causes intense, burning pain locally or throughout the body. Then painful and intensely itchy cross-hatching lines of red bumps and welts crop up wherever nematocysts contact skin. These tentacle tracks may blister, bleed, ulcerate, become hyperpigmented, and leave permanent scars. Severe envenomations may cause nausea and vomiting, weakness, anxiety, sweating, vertigo, runny eyes and nose, shortness of breath, headache, muscle spasms, kidney failure, a sense of impending doom, shock, and (rarely) death.

Jellyfish

Myriad jellyfish populate Atlantic (the Chesapeake Bay *sea nettle, moon jelly, cabbage-head jellyfish*), Caribbean (*sea wasp, jimble*), and Pacific (*purple-striped stinger*) coastal waters and have the same basic shape as the Portuguese man-of-war. But instead of a gas-filled sail which floats on the surface, jellyfish have a bell which floats below the surface and from which hang up to twelve hundred tentacles. The bells range in size from less than an inch to more than 6 feet, and the tentacles often exceed 120 feet in length. The tentacles may be colored or transparent. Like the Portuguese man-of-war, jellyfish are swept along by wind and current, using their tentacles to find and kill prey.

Jellyfish venom is among the most potent toxins known. *Chironex fleckeri*, the dreaded box-jellyfish, is the most venomous marine animal. Its sting can kill a man in 30 seconds. Fortunately, it's found only off the coast of northern Australia and in western Indo-Pacific waters. Jellyfish stings generally cause a severe, stinging, burning pain and scattered bumps, wheals, or cross-hatched lines of welts on the skin. Stings of the eye can cause corneal ulcerations. Serious envenomations may cause muscle spasms, vomiting, dizziness, confusion, chest pain, headache, shock, and nightmares. Some people become sensitized to jellyfish and have serious allergic reactions that may include wheezing, airway swelling, shock, and collapse.

Sea Anemones and Corals

Sea anemones are coelenterates, but they look like colored flowers. They grow on coral reefs and in shallow tidal pools, where they sting swimmers and waders who brush up against their nematocyst-armed tentacles. Their sting is mild, but they produce a rash that can become ulcerated and infected.

The ancients held that *stony corals* had the power to ward off lightning, whirlwind, shipwreck, and fire. I don't know about that, but the pointed horns and razor-sharp edges of the animal's calcareous outer skeleton can shred the skin of a diver. The cuts and abrasions cause minor burning pain, and itchy, red wheals appear but fade after an hour or two. This reaction is called "coral poisoning." The wounds may blister, or become infected, ulcerate, and slough, and take up to six weeks to heal.

Treatment
Vigorously scrub coral cuts with soap and water. Then irrigate the wounds with a forceful jet of fresh water using a syringe and nee-

dle. If the wounds sting, rinse them with dilute (5%) vinegar or 40 to 70% isopropyl alcohol to deactivate nematocysts. Large lacerations should be packed open or loosely closed with tape closures.

Treatment of Coelenterate Envenomations

1. Remove tentacles with gloved hands or instruments.

2. Rinse the skin with lots of salt water. (CAUTION: Fresh water and rubbing will trigger the nematocysts.)

3. Deactivate the nematocysts by soaking the exposed skin in a dilute vinegar solution for 30 minutes or until the stinging stops. Use 40 to 70% isopropyl alcohol or Stingose if you don't have vinegar. Meat tenderizer destroys the venom; if you have any, throw a few pinches into the vinegar or alcohol. Cover sea nettle stings with a baking soda slurry for 10 minutes, and then scrape it off.

4. Remove the remaining nematocysts by applying shaving cream to the area and scraping the skin with a razor. Or make a paste with mud, flour, or talc and scrape it off with a sharpened shell or knife.

5. Gently dry the skin, and apply Solarcaine, Itch Balm Plus, Benadryl cream or 1% hydrocortisone ointment.

6. Take diphenhydramine, 50 mg every 6 hours, for mild allergic reactions.

7. Movement causes the venom to spread, so immobilize the injured part and keep it elevated above heart level.

8. Cleanse ulcerating wounds with antiseptic solution every 6 hours and cover them with sterile dressings.

9. Serious envenomations and life-threatening allergic reactions require emergency medical attention. An antivenin to the box-jellyfish is available from the Commonwealth Serum Laboratories of Australia.

ECHINODERMS

Three classes of venomous animals in this phylum cause human grief.

Crown of Thorns Starfish

This large (up to 2 feet) starfish is found in the Indo-Pacific area and in the eastern Pacific from the Galapagos to the Gulf of California. The surface of this animal is covered with sharp, venom-tipped spines that inflict painful wounds, bleeding, and swelling. Multiple stings can cause nausea, vomiting, swollen lymph nodes, numbness, and paralysis.

Treatment

Immerse the wounded part in hot water (110 to 115 degrees Fahrenheit) until the pain dissipates; then irrigate the wound and remove foreign debris.

Sea Urchins

Sea urchins are the porcupines of the sea. They are elongated or ball-shaped creatures that are covered with long, sharp, and brittle spines that often break off after puncturing the hide of a snorkeler or diver. Some of these spines carry venom, and small pincers (pedicellariae) scattered among the spines grab onto prey and continue to bite and inject venom as long as the victim moves. Most sea urchin injuries are the result of a diver or swimmer stepping onto or brushing against the animal. The spines penetrate deep into the flesh and cause immediate hellish, burning pain, redness, swelling, and bleeding. Multiple spine punctures may cause nausea, numbness, weakness, abdominal pain, paralysis, difficulty breathing, fainting, muscle and joint pains, and (rarely) shock and death. One or two months after the original injury, a *granuloma* (round, fleshy mass) or diffuse inflammation at the wound site may appear.

Treatment

1. Immerse the injured part in 110 to 115 degree Fahrenheit water for 30 to 60 minutes.

2. Remove embedded spines carefully. Spines that puncture joints, nerves, or tendons must be removed surgically as soon as possible. If left in the tissues, spines can cause deep infections and granulomas. (The body will resorb a thin spine in 3 to 8 weeks; you can leave an inaccessible thin spine alone if it hasn't entered a joint or impinged on nerves or blood vessels.)

3. Cleanse the wound thoroughly with antiseptic solution.

4. If the wound is deep, take TMP-SMX or ciprofloxacin twice daily for 2 days to ward off infection.

Sea Cucumbers

These sausage-shaped bottom dwellers are found in all the seas of the world, in deep or shallow waters. They can envenom you with their own toxin (*holothurin*) or with the coelenterate venom they extract from munching on nematocysts. You may get mild skin irritation after handling a sea cucumber, or severe conjunctivitis or corneal inflammation if your eyes are exposed to the toxin.

Treatment
Bathe the exposed skin in dilute vinegar or isopropyl alcohol. Eye injuries should be evaluated by an ophthalmologist as soon as possible.

BRISTLEWORMS

The ocean floor is crawling with segmented marine worms. The bristleworm and other species have tiny bristles on their foot parts that can penetrate human skin and cause a painful, hivelike red rash.

Treatment
Remove embedded bristles with tweezers or adhesive tape. Then rinse the affected area with dilute vinegar or isopropyl alcohol.

CONE SHELLS

Cone shells are attractive, beautifully colored killers. These venomous mollusks are found in shallow waters, tide pools, and reefs off the coasts of Hawaii, Mexico, and California. They burrow in the sand or coral during the day and emerge at night to kill prey with a venomous, barbed proboscis. Most cone shell victims are divers or swimmers who pick up the shell and get stung on the hand. A burning sting is followed by transient disruption of blood flow to the area, bluish discoloration, and numbness. Serious envenomations cause tingling in the area of the wound that spreads to the lips and then the entire body. Some victims have difficulty speaking and swallowing, weakness, itching, blurred and double vision, loss of consciousness, brain swelling, coma, and death due to heart failure. Generalized muscle paralysis may lead to respiratory arrest and death.

Treatment

1. Immerse the injured part in hot water (110 to 115 degrees Fahrenheit) until pain is relieved. (Heat may partially inactivate the venom.)

2. Apply a pressure bandage over the sting site and secure it with elastic bandages. This may help retard movement of the venom into the general circulation. The bandage should be tight enough to occlude the veins and lymph channels, but not so tight as to impede inflow of arterial blood to the extremity. Check the pulses below the bandage periodically, and loosen the bandage if they are weak or absent, or if the digits turn blue and cold. Keep the pressure bandage on until you arrive at a medical facility.

3. Clean and irrigate the wound and cover it with a sterile dressing.

Prevention

1. Wear gloves when handling cone shells.

2. Drop the shell like a hot potato if the proboscis protrudes.

3. Collectors should use a bucket to gather the shells; divers would be wise not to carry them inside their wet suit.

•
•
•
•
•

18

SHARKS AND
OTHER MARINE MARAUDERS

*When his head was almost upon me, his jaw plainly
visible beneath, I brought my fist down across my body and
managed to hit him on the eyes, the nose. The flesh was torn
from my left arm. He passed me and as he did so I could feel
the movement of his great body against me.*

*"My whole mind and body now centered on the battle
against annihilation, as if I were an animal fighting off a
stronger, larger beast. . . . Each time he attacked on the
surface I could hit him, but each time he took another nip
out of me. After an attack I would raise my feet and arms
to see what I had left. The big toe on my left foot was
dangling. A piece of my right heel was gone. My left elbow,
hand and calf were torn. If he did not actually sink his teeth
into me, his rough hide would scrape off great pieces of my
skin. The salt water stanched the flow of blood somewhat
and I was not conscious of great pain. The physical shock of
the encounter served to keep that in check for a while.*

—Lieutenant Commander Herbert Kabat,
as quoted by Edward E. Leslie,
Desperate Journeys, Abandoned Souls

SHARKS

Statistically, shark attacks are rare occurrences; only fifty to a
hundred are reported worldwide each year. You are much more
likely to be struck by lightning than to be attacked by a shark.
Nevertheless, shark attacks are memorable events for those, like
Commander Kabat, who survive them.

Sharks have been cruising the oceans of the world for 375 million years. They have changed very little in that time, a testament
to their proficiency at finding and killing prey and fighting off

competitors. Of the three hundred and fifty or so shark species, only thirty-two are known people-eaters. These include some of the bigger sharks, such as the great white, mako, hammerhead, grey reef, blue, dusky, and bull sharks. The basking shark, on the other hand, which grows to 40 feet, is so docile that my fishermen on the Aran Islands once hunted them in curraghs.

Some shark species venture into fresh water. The bull shark regularly swims up the rivers of Florida's west coast and has been found in Lake Okeechobee. He also thrives in the fresh water of Lake Nicaragua in Central America, where he terrorizes the native population.

The great white shark, popularized by fiction writers and Hollywood in recent years, is a real brute. In 1978, a 29-foot 6-inch, 10,000-pound great white was harpooned and landed in the Azores. Fortunately, most great whites aren't that large, but they are aggressive. They are implicated in more attacks on humans than any other shark species, many of these attacks taking place off the east coast of Australia, the South African coast near Durban, off the mid-Atlantic coast of the United States, and north of Point Conception, California.

The tiger shark, which can grow to a length of 18 feet and may weigh up to a ton, is another heavyweight with a taste for humans. The great hammerhead shark's fearsome appearance reinforces his reputation as a man-eater in tropical waters.

The Setting

Sharks prefer warm water, and most attacks occur in a band from 46 degrees north latitude to 47 degrees south latitude. Sharks are more likely to attack during the late afternoon and evening (when they actively feed) and in warm (70 degrees Fahrenheit), murky waters. Great whites tolerate cooler waters and have been implicated in a number of human attacks in recent years off the northern California coast.

When career bank robber Willie Sutton was asked why he robbed banks, he replied, "Because that's where the money is." Most reported shark attacks occur within 100 feet of shore, because that's where the people are. But the danger of shark attack is statistically much greater in coastal estuaries, deep channels, and drop-offs, all prime shark habitats.

Sharks, like most piscine predators, are attracted to movement, contrasting colors, and bright or reflecting objects. They have been known to scarf down surfers paddling out to catch "the big wave," presumably taking them to be elephant seals, a shark delicacy.

Shark Physiology 101

Sharks aren't exceptionally bright, but they have other talents. Their keen sense of smell enables them to detect blood, urine, and peritoneal fluid in parts per billion, and those cold, soulless eyes quickly perceive and lock onto any motion in the water. A shark's lateral-line organs and sensors in the ampullae of Lorenzini near his head can detect vibrations and low-frequency sounds miles distant, enabling him to home in on a struggling fish or a swimmer in distress.

Shark Psychology 101

No one really knows what motivates a beast as primal as the shark, but animal behaviorists believe that he is stimulated to attack either by hunger or by a threat to his territory or mating area. Since the majority of shark-attack victims are bitten only once or twice, in most attacks the shark is probably just trying to scare the transgressor off. Before making a territorial attack, some sharks arch their backs, stiffen their bodies, and waggle their tails (see Figure 27). That's your exit cue. If you hang around, your next warning might be a solitary upper tooth slash (sharks generally use their bottom teeth first when feeding).

Dum-dum, Dum-dum, Dum-dum: The Attack

A shark's motives are of more than academic interest to a swimmer who suddenly sees a sinister dorsal fin slicing through the water.

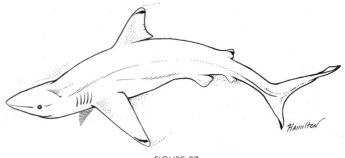

FIGURE 27
Shark's warning posture.

A shark that is defending his territory may only give a warning nip. A feeding shark, on the other hand, strikes suddenly, violently, and with all the fury of a kamikaze. It swims with deceptively graceful, languid movements of its body and tail as it slowly closes in on its prey in ever-tightening circles. It may deliver a "bump" first, presumably to wound and immobilize its victim. (This bump is no love tap, and the shark's shagreen, or skin, so coarse and abrasive it was once used by sailors to holystone the decks of sailing ships, can cause massive, deep abrasions.) When the shark moves in for the kill, it puts on a burst of speed, tilts its head slightly backward, advances its upper jaw, and slams its granite-hard, razor-sharp teeth deep into its victim's flesh. Then it shakes its head back and forth, like a terrier shaking a rat, and rips away a limb or a hunk of flesh. The bite leaves a mutilating, crescent-shaped wound, with both crush injuries and massive avulsions of tissue. Large sharks, whose jaws have a biting force of up to 18 tons per square inch, can snap a man in half with one violent bite.

If other sharks are attracted to the scene, the swimmer or diver will be the *pièce de résistance* in a shark feeding frenzy. In a feeding frenzy a gang of sharks, excited by the smell of blood and flesh, goes berserk and savagely attacks everything in sight, including each other, until the sea becomes a boiling, red caldron.

The Aftermath

Sharks have rows of jagged, razor-sharp teeth embedded in huge, crescent-shaped jaws. Armed with such fearsome dentition and pile driver jaws, they easily shred bone, muscle, blood vessels, tendons, and viscera, creating grievous wounds. The victim's arms and legs are bitten most often, and are often snapped off. Bites of the chest or abdominal cavity are usually fatal. Many shark-attack victims exsanguinate within moments of being attacked, while others are disabled and drown. But most victims are bitten only once or twice, and if they are removed from the water and their bleeding is controlled quickly enough, they may live to tell about their ordeal.

Treatment

Shock from massive blood loss is the usual cause of death from shark attack. Combat shock by firmly applying large compresses to bleeding wounds, while the victim is still in the water if possible. If there is a medically trained person on board, he or she should ligate (tie off) any arterial bleeders that can't be controlled with firm compression and start intravenous fluids if the necessary supplies are at hand. If direct compression and ligation don't control bleeding, tourniquets may be lifesaving (see Chapter 1).

While you are rendering lifesaving first aid, keep the patient warm and arrange for immediate evacuation to a hospital.

Prevention

• Don't swim in shark-infested waters, and don't swim or dive in murky waters, deep channels, or drop-offs; near sewage outflow tracts; or in areas where fish or animal scraps are dumped.

• Don't swim in known shark-infested waters with domestic animals. Stories abound of sharks attacking land animals of all kinds, from dogs and cats to cattle, horses, and elephants.

• Avoid swimming at dusk or in the evening when sharks are hungriest.

• Sharks are more likely to attack a lone swimmer, so swim in groups, and stay alert. If a shark shows up, move slowly out of the water, and try not to act scared.

• If a shark approaches while you are diving, resist the urge to blast out of the water like a Trident missile. Instead, move to a defensive position on the bottom, or against a cliff or rock formation.

• You may be able to deflect a charging shark with a sharp rap to the snout or a poke in the gills or eyes. Or you may be able to spook him by directing a stream of bubbles from your regulator in his direction.

• Some of the old adventure movies depicted the hero engaging in hand-to-fin combat with a shark and killing him with a knife after a prolonged and thrilling underwater struggle. Don't you try to do that. The shark has the home-field advantage, and all the commotion will just arouse the curiosity of other sharks and trigger a feeding frenzy. You may win the battle but lose the war.

• Stay out of the water if you have an open wound or are menstruating, and don't urinate in the water.

• Be alert for sharks when schools of fish start to act squirrely.

• If you are spearfishing, trail your catch on a long tether. If you attach them to your belt, you may as well wear a bull's-eye.

• Don't wear brightly colored swimsuits or shiny diving or snorkeling gear.

• Don't deliberately provoke sharks. (If you enjoy teasing sharks, you have a death wish.)

• Swim with regular, smooth strokes. The sound of splashing and surface commotion is a dinner gong to a shark.

• Don't rely on shark repellents. They don't work.

BARRACUDA

We arrived . . . just in time to take on board one of my boys, who had been badly bitten by a barracuda. . . . This lad while fishing on his own in a small rowboat, had caught a four-foot barracuda, and dumped it in the bow without taking the trouble to kill it. Not long afterward . . . the boy reached back of him for some bait. The barracuda threw itself from its position some distance away on the bottom of the boat and fastened its cruel, lacerating teeth in the boy's right forearm, making a horrible wound. . . . I had never before known any sort of sea creature to jump and bite a man except when both were in the water, and it gave me a new conception of this fish's weapons.

—Captain William E. Young, *Shark! Shark!*

I wouldn't want to get into a *boat* with a fish like the *great barracuda*, much less the water. This is a fish with an attitude, a savage, fearless and inquisitive denizen of tropical waters. Despite its smaller size (4 to 5 feet on average, although some monsters grow to 10 feet), Caribbean natives fear the great barracuda more than they fear sharks. He seldom attacks swimmers or divers, but when he does, he strikes like a torpedo with teeth, long, lancet-like teeth in two parallel rows that can rip and tear flesh with savage efficiency. Barracuda seem to be enraged by bright, reflecting objects, and one of the surest ways to get bitten by one of these toothy fish is to dangle your arms or legs over the side of a boat, especially if they are adorned with shiny jewelry.

Treatment
Barracuda bites create straight or V-shaped wounds which present all of the problems of shark bites, although on a smaller scale. As in shark bites, first aid consists of controlling hemorrhage and getting the victim to a hospital ASAP.

Prevention
• Keep your arms and legs out of the water when cruising tropical waters.
• Don't swim or dive in turbid water. (Barracuda become confused and antsy in murky water.)
• Don't wear reflective jewelry while swimming or diving; avoid sudden movements.

• Avoid surface splashing, which will draw barracuda to you like a magnet.

• Keep captured fish on a long tether while diving if you don't want to lose your love handles to a ravenous barracuda.

MORAY EELS

Eels are those slimy, snakelike fish that slither along the bottom and that are nearly impossible to get off your fishhook. The moray eel is a little bigger than most eels, and a lot more dangerous. Only sharks make more attacks on humans. It has a heavy, compact body, and its skin is thick, leathery, and spotted (see Figure 28). The back of its head is elevated, he has small, round gill openings on its snout, and its powerful, viselike jaws are studded with long, sharp, retrorse teeth. It looks like a creature that lives in a hole, and he does. Either a hole or some dark crevice on the sea bottom.

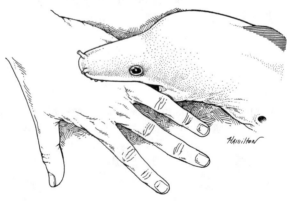

FIGURE 28
Moray eel biting hand of diver.

Morays have been around since the Pleistocene era (at least two million years), and were well known to the ancients. Hircius, a well-to-do Roman, kept a reservoir filled with six thousand morays to serve at banquets for the emperor. Another Roman,

Vedius Pollio, communicated his displeasure to insubordinate slaves by tossing them into his moray tank, sending them to a horrible death with the words, "Ad muraenas!" (The Romans believed that a steady diet of humans made moray meat tastier.)

Moray eels inhabit rocky coral reefs in tropical and temperate waters on the east coast of North America from New Jersey to Yucatan, Mexico, and on the west coast from Baja California to Point Conception.

The moray's forbidding countenance belies his shy, retiring temperament. He generally won't attack unless he is cornered or provoked. But a moray's hole is his castle, and when a curious diver sticks his hand into that hole, the moray drops his Dr. Jekyll persona and assumes the vicious character of a Mr. Hyde. He buries his fanglike teeth in the hapless diver's hand and hangs on with the ferocity and tenacity of a bulldog. Nothing short of decapitation or jaw disarticulation with pliers or a crowbar can loosen the moray's grip on that hand. The resulting wound is a series of deep punctures that can damage nerves, muscles, joints, tendons, and blood vessels. And the moray's long teeth drive marine bacteria deep into the tissues, so serious infection is a common complication of moray bites.

Treatment

1. First, remove the moray from the victim. (You may need a large, ultrasharp knife and a tool kit to do that.)

2. Use direct pressure to control bleeding.

3. Remove broken teeth and other debris from the wound.

4. Cleanse superficial wounds with antiseptic solution.

5. Use a syringe and a 20-gauge needle to thoroughly irrigate the puncture wounds with sterile saline solution (if available) or disinfected water.

6. Don't close lacerations; leave them open so that they can drain if they become infected. Simply apply a thin layer of antibiotic ointment and cover the wound with sterile dressings.

7. Give the victim TMP-SMX, one tablet every 12 hours, as wound infection prophylaxis.

Prevention

I would no sooner put my hand into a hole or rocky crevice on the sea bottom than I would put it into a garbage disposal unit. Keep your hands out of his hole, and the moray will keep his teeth out of your hand.

GROUPERS

Giant groupers are big tropical fish that divers often try to hitch a ride on. They look like giant bass and range up to 12 feet in length and 1,000 pounds in weight. And like all big animals, they are prodigious eaters. (Some biblical scholars speculate that Jonah wasn't swallowed by a whale, but was scarfed down by a hungry grouper when he was thrown overboard.)

Groupers aren't especially aggressive, but they aren't shy either and they become feisty when defending their territory. The bite of their powerful jaws produces a ragged crush injury, with a great deal of soft-tissue damage.

Treatment

Grouper bites are treated like shark and barracuda bites. The hand is a favorite target of groupers. To control pain and swelling, keep it elevated and iced for at least 48 hours after it is cleansed and bandaged.

Prevention

Groupers like to lurk in shipwrecks and caves. Take a good look around places like this before entering so that you don't disturb a slumbering grouper. If he tries to escape, don't get in his way. And carry speared fish on a long tether.

•
•
•
•
•

19

LIGHTNING ON THE HIGH SEAS

*The terrible clap of thunder slew four of our men outright,
their necks being wrung in sunder without speaking any
word. Of our 94 men there was not one untouched. Some
were struck blind, others bruised in legs and arms. Some
were bruised in their breasts so they voided blood two days
after. Still others were drawn out at length, as if they had
been racked, but all recovered, save the four.*

—Sir James Lancaster of the Royal Navy,
*The Voyages of Sir James Lancaster to Brazil
and the East Indies, 1591–1603*

The lightning that struck this British vessel off Cape Corrientes
in 1591 splintered the mainmast and melted iron spikes 10 inches
within the timber. Such lightning-wrought devastation was an
accepted hazard for Royal Navy ships before the advent of marine
lightning conductors in the late eighteenth century. Until that
time, an untold number of ships had been lost, destroyed by fire,
or disabled by lightning, and innumerable sailors injured or killed.
Which is hardly surprising when you consider that there are fifty
thousand thunderstorms and eight million lightning strikes each
day throughout the world.

The sulphurous, gunpowderlike smell that hangs in the air after
a lightning strike led our maritime forebears to conclude that its
destructive effects were due to some sort of explosion. It wasn't
until 1752 that Benjamin Franklin enticed a few sparks of electricity out of the end of a kite string, proving that lightning was just
a giant electric spark. This discovery paved the way for the inven-
tion and adoption of marine lightning conductors.

GENERATOR IN THE SKY

But what *causes* lightning? The Vikings believed that thunder and lightning was Thor's Hammer *Mjolnir* hurtling through the heavens. The ancient Akkadians believed that lightning bolts were created when the weather god cracked his whip at the horses pulling his chariot. The early Greeks held that lightning bolts were hurled from the sky by angry gods:

> *Then Zeus let fly his thunderbolts, and the ship went round and round, and was filled with fire and brimstone as the lightning struck it.*

> —Homer, *The Odyssey*

Modern atmospheric scientists subscribe to this scenario.

1. When a cold front collides with a warm front, warm, moist air rises into the upper atmosphere, forming a cumulonimbus cloud. When high winds flatten the top of the cloud, it becomes the classic anvil-shaped thundercloud.

2. The warm, moist air cools and forms ice particles, and enormous electric charges accumulate as these particles collide with one another in the powerful updrafts and downdrafts. A net positive charge accumulates in the upper regions of the cloud, a net negative charge in the lower regions.

3. Air, being a poor conductor of electricity, insulates and separates areas of opposite charge within the cloud until the potential difference reaches hundreds of millions of volts. At that point, the air becomes a conductor, and an electric current of 10,000 to 20,000 amps flashes from one region of the cloud to another in the form of *sheet* lightning.

4. The negative charge in the bottom of the cloud induces a positive charge on the ground below.

5. A lightning strike is initiated by a *leader stroke* that moves from the cloud toward the ground. (This is a relatively slow-moving (1 million cm/sec) stroke carrying a charge of up to 3,000,000 volts and a current of 250,000 amps.)

6. A *pilot stroke* rises from the ground, a mast, an antenna, or some other structure, meets the leader stroke, and the two strokes create a channel of ions, a low-resistance pathway between ground and cloud. A much more rapid (1 billion cm/sec) and powerful *return stroke* surges from the ground to the cloud along this pathway, heats the channel to more than 50,000 degrees Fahrenheit, and equalizes the potential difference between cloud and ground, which peaks at several hundred million volts.

Enormous energy is required to overcome air resistance and create an ion channel, so the leader stroke is the brightest and most visible of the sequence of strokes. That and its relative slowness make it the most visible of the strokes, creating the illusion that lightning is traveling from cloud to ground. In fact, it's the return stroke that channels the bulk of the energy in the opposite direction. But it moves too fast to be seen.

St. Elmo's Fire

Upon the maintopgallant mast-head, was a ball of light,
which the sailors call a corposant (corpus sancti), and which
the mate had called out to us to look at . . . for sailors have
a notion that if the corposant rises in the rigging it is a sign of
fair weather, but if it comes lower down there will be a
storm.

—Richard Henry Dana, *Two Years Before the Mast*

St. Elmo's fire, the eerie pale blue or green light sometimes seen in a ship's rigging, is static electricity induced by a thunder cloud. (Sailors of old feared "the Fire," and called it, variously, "Castor and Pollux," "the corposants," "Sailor Devil," "Corbie's Aunt," "Helen's Fire," or "Davy Jones.")

Thunder

According to nautical legend, thunder is the sound of Henry Hudson's crew playing tenpins in Fiddler's Green. Could be, but it's more likely to represent shock waves created by the explosive expansion of superheated air around a lightning strike. Low, rumbling thunder comes from a distant lightning strike; a sharp crack means the strike was nearby and you'd better get cracking yourself. (You can estimate your distance from a lightning strike by counting the time between strike and thunder in seconds. Distance in miles equals seconds divided by 5.)

Different Strokes for Different Folks

Streak lightning is the classic, forked lightning bolt. But lightning takes other forms as well, including:

1. *Sheet lightning,* a formless flash of current between two clouds, sometimes seen above the horizon.

2. *Bead lightning,* caused by lingering areas of ionization and charge in the afterstrokes.

3. *Ribbon lightning,* streak lightning deformed by high winds.

4. *Ball lightning,* an eerie, grapefruit-sized luminescent ball of electrical energy whose behavior is unpredictable. During a thunderstorm in 1685, a "ball of fire" floated into a gun room aboard the HMS *Coronation,* knocked a boy overboard, rendered several workmen unconscious, scorched timbers, and broke glass windows before dispersing itself on the deck. In 1749, a "ball of fire" skimmed over the surface of the sea until it reached HMS *Montague,* then rose vertically above the main chains of the bowsprit. It exploded, knocking down five men, and badly burning one of them, and shattered the mainmast and the main topmast.

Blitzkrieg ("Lightning War")

The open water is one of the most dangerous places to be during a thunderstorm. It's hard to keep your mind on fishing, sailing, or waterskiing when those menacing, black thunderclouds start moving your way, with lightning flashing in the wings and thunder booming like cosmic artillery.

Lightning is attracted to the highest object, and if that happens to be your boat, it will strike the mast, the fly bridge, a metal antenna, or you, and take the path of least resistance to the water. That path may involve detours through your plumbing and electrical systems. It can rupture hoses and fracture PVC connectors leading into bronze seacocks. And the electromagnetic pulse associated with lightning can damage the diodes in your engine's alternator and reverse the polarity of your compass.

The "Cone of Protection"

If your boat is well-grounded, a "cone of protection" projects down at an angle of 60 degrees from the masthead or superstructure to a circle at water level having a radius approximately equal to the height of the mast (see figure 29). This cone of protection confers a probability of protection of 99.0 percent. Raising the mast so that the apex angle of the cone is 45 degrees will increase the probability of protection to 99.9 percent.

A marine lightning conductor or ground consists of No. 8 gauge wire leading from the masthead straight to a porous bronze grounding plate attached to the hull below the water line. (Any submerged metal surface at least 1 foot in area, such as the propeller, a radio ground plate, or a metal rudder, will serve as a ground

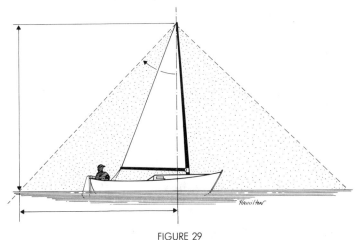

FIGURE 29
Cone of protection around sailboat with lightning conductor in mast.

connection.) Additional leads should run from spot lights, deck railings, the engine block, 110-watt shore power, and any large metal objects within the hull or superstructure to the conductor. Metal standing rigging on a sailboat should be bonded together and connected to the ground. Tall radio antennas that are fitted with transmitting-type lightning arresters or are connected to ground act as lightning rods and will confer a cone of protection on a powerboat. Fiberglass whip antennas don't conduct electricity and offer no protection against lightning.

If your boat isn't grounded, you can jury-rig a ground by attaching a jumper cable to the highest point on the boat and trailing the other end in the water.

LIGHTNING INJURY

When Poseidon throws that lightning bolt, you'd better duck, because lightning kills 30 percent of its victims and maims two-thirds of the survivors.

Mechanisms of Injury

Lightning injuries can result from:

1. *Direct strike,* if you aren't in a cone of protection.

2. *Contact* with an object that is struck, such as a railing or mast.

3. *Flash discharge* (*"splash"*), as lightning jumps from the struck object to you.

4. *Ground current,* if you're swimming when lightning strikes the boat.

The "Flashover Effect"

A lightning bolt has much greater amperage and voltage than commercial electricity. But unlike commercial electricity, which penetrates the skin and causes internal injuries, lightning strike is nearly instantaneous, and contact with the skin is too brief to allow penetration. Instead, the current flows over the outside of the body, vaporizes moisture on the skin, and sometimes blows the victim's shoes and socks off! This conduction of the current over the surface of the body is called "flashover." (Samuel Pepys told of a Genoese galley slave who had his leg shackle melted off by a bolt of lightning. His leg was uninjured, but the poor wretch was immediately reshackled.)

Specific Injuries

• *Cardiopulmonary.* Flashover saves most lightning victims. But lightning can act like a massive cosmic countershock, causing cardiac standstill and paralyzing the respiratory center in the brain. The heart quickly resumes beating, but the respiratory center takes longer to recover. After going without oxygen for a few minutes, the heart fibrillates (*secondary cardiac arrest*) and the victim dies. Although "struck dead," these people are eminently savable if CPR is started during the "golden period" between cardiac standstill and secondary cardiac arrest.

• *Central nervous system.* Getting struck in the head by lightning is like getting beaned with a cosmic belaying pin. It can fracture the skull, cause massive scalp bleeding and epidural and subdural hematomas, and coagulate the gray matter. Most lightning victims suffer loss of consciousness, temporary paralysis of the arms or legs, and amnesia. Many have transient or persistent seizures, headaches, mood disturbances, intellectual impairment, insomnia, and lightning phobia for months afterward.

• *Eyes.* Lightning can cause temporary blindness, retinal detachment, bleeding into the front or back chamber of the eye, double vision, sensitivity to light, loss of color vision, and degeneration of the optic nerves. The pupils may be widely dilated and unresponsive to light for a while after the lightning strike. (Fixed and dilated pupils are generally a reliable sign of brain death, but should not be so construed in a lightning victim.)

• *Ears.* At ground zero, thunder sounds like two aircraft carriers colliding head-on at flank speed. The sound and shock wave of a lightning strike can rupture the eardrums and cause temporary deafness, vertigo, and impaired balance.

• *Skin.* As that 14,000-degree thunderbolt flashes over the outside of the body, it produces a variety of burns, including *linear burns* on the head, chest, and legs where sweat vaporizes into steam; clusters of *punctate burns* that look like cigarette burns; superficial *feathering burns* ("ferning") caused by the imprint of electron showers; and second- or third-degree burns caused by superheated jewelry, coins, or belt buckles.

• *Circulation.* Spasm of blood vessels results in mottled, cool extremities and diminished or absent pulses. The spasm generally subsides after a few hours.

• *Muscles and bones.* Lightning strike causes violent, sustained muscle contractions that can produce fractures, dislocations, and spine injuries.

• *Blast.* Lightning's explosive force can cause head injury, fractures, spinal injury, internal bleeding, rib fractures, lung contusion, and ruptured abdominal organs.

Treatment

The HMS *Sir Francis Drake* was struck by lightning off Java in 1806. The thirteen men who were on deck at the time were resuscitated "by inflation of their lungs, by friction to their bare skin, and by throwing buckets of water over them."

The *Drake*'s doctor knew something about lightning injuries. "Inflation of the lungs" is precisely the correct treatment for a person apparently "struck dead" by lightning. Seventy percent of these people can be resuscitated if they receive CPR (see Chapter 1).

Sorting Things Out

If lightning strikes your ungrounded boat, all those on deck will very likely get zapped as the lightning "splashes" from the mast or superstructure. The standard approach to mass casualties is to *triage* ("sort") the victims into three categories, and treat them in this order:

1. Those who will live if they are treated immediately.

2. Those who will live whether they are treated or not.

3. Those who are going to die no matter what is done for them.

If your deck is strewn with lightning casualties, you should first "resuscitate the dead," and then attend the others. Victims who are moaning may be badly hurt, but at least they are breathing. Disregard them until you resuscitate and stabilize those who are in cardiac or respiratory arrest (no spontaneous breathing, with or without pulses). If you perform CPR during the golden period between cardiac standstill and secondary cardiac arrest, you may number among your crew a modern-day Lazarus.

Back to the ABCs

Approach the lightning victim as you would any multiple trauma victim. Follow the ABCs (Airway, Breathing, and Circulation, see Chapter 1) and you won't go wrong. Remember, the violent tetanic contractions triggered by lightning strike can cause spinal injuries, long-bone fractures, and dislocations. Keep the neck immobilized at all times, and splint suspected fractures or dislocations. Move the victim into the cabin as soon as you can do so safely, and continue evaluation and treatment there. Once he has resumed breathing, remove his clothing and do a head-to-toe exam.

• *Head.* Look for signs of trauma: scalp burns or cuts, bleeding or drainage of clear fluid from the nose or ears, amnesia, confusion, perseveration (repeating the same questions over and over), loose teeth, or facial fractures.

• *Eyes, Ears, and Nose.* Check the size and reactivity of the pupils, visual acuity (have him count fingers or read print), and eye movement. Look for blood in the front of the eye and embedded foreign bodies. Check the hearing, and examine the eardrum by pulling the outer ear up and back while shining a light into the ear canal (bleeding may represent a ruptured drum or a basilar skull fracture). Check for nosebleeds.

• *Spine.* Check for tenderness and deformity by running your fingers down the tips of the spines from the base of the scalp to the tailbone. Check for fractures by lightly thumping the spine with your fist.

• *Chest.* Observe, listen, and feel for signs of chest injuries. Listen to the heart tones; are they clear and regular?

• *Abdomen.* Is it soft, or is it distended, rigid, and tender? Can you hear bowel sounds?

• *Pelvis and extremities.* Check the pulses at the wrists, groin, and feet, and look for paralysis, deformities, crepitus, tenderness, and open fractures. Check the color, warmth, motion, and sensation of the toes and fingers.

• *Skin.* Look for burns and mottling.

Treat injuries according to the instructions in Chapters 1 to 6. If the victim is unconscious, confused, or hypotensive, and you can start an intravenous line, 0.9% normal saline or Ringer's lactate are the fluids of choice. Infuse the solution at 125 cc an hour, or more rapidly if the patient is hypotensive or in shock. Most lightning burns are superficial and need no treatment. Treat deeper burns as described in Chapter 2. Ruptured eardrums require no special treatment unless contaminated with foreign matter, in which case you should give amoxicillin, 250 mg three times a day for 7 to 10 days.

All lightning victims should ideally be evaluated and treated in a hospital as soon as possible. If you are in mid-ocean, do the best you can with the resources at your disposal, keeping in mind that many lightning injuries, including concussion, paralysis, deafness, blindness, and burns, will resolve over time.

Prevention

What do you do if you're out in your boat and you see ominous thunderheads forming in the distance? The answer depends on where you are, your boat's hull construction, and whether it is grounded. The best option is to head for shore, if you think you can beat the storm. If you're offshore, and there's a bigger boat with a tall mast in the area, pull alongside and take advantage of its cone of protection. Empty your pockets of metal objects, take off any jewelry or belt buckles, stay away from the mast and shrouds, pump the bilge, and stay in the cabin. Don't touch electrical appliances or equipment, radio antennas or lead-in wires, or any grounded metal object. Be especially careful that you don't bridge two such objects by touching both at the same time. And stay out of the head; people have been blown off the seat by lightning passing through water-filled hoses leading to through-hull fittings!

If your sailboat has a wire lifting bridle, you can turn it into an emergency lightning conductor by wrapping it around the shrouds and dropping the end over the side and into the water.

If you're in an aluminum boat, you're sitting in a floating lightning rod. You are at high risk for a direct strike; you may also be injured by ground current if lightning strikes the water anywhere within 100 yards.

Fiberglass is a poor conductor of electricity and doesn't attract lightning. But fiberglass boats can act as giant capacitors. If the occupants pick up a positive charge from a thundercloud, the fiberglass hull prevents this charge from being conducted into the water (ground). If the potential difference between occupants and water becomes great enough, there will be a powerful discharge of electric current through the boat, shocking and possibly killing those on board.

If you are swimming, get out of the water immediately. If you are on a beach, stay low until the storm lets up. If you are on a sailboard, let the mast and sail down and lie down on the board.

Fishing rods, especially graphite and boron rods, can act as lightning rods. Reel in those lines at the first sign of a thunderstorm.

20
A SHIP'S MEDICINE CHEST

You know about Murphy's Law, but have you heard of Gill's Corollary to Murphy's Law? It goes like this: Any sickness or injury that *can* happen ashore, *will* happen at sea.

No cruising veteran would dispute the immutability of Gill's Corollary. Nor would he put to sea without a well-stocked medical kit with which to treat the sprains, bruises, cuts, seasickness, sunburn, and headaches which are an inevitable part of every cruise.

I wouldn't think of pulling away from the dock without a medical kit on board. The one I keep on my boat contains an assortment of wound-care materials, splints, elastic bandages, medications, tweezers, scissors, and miscellanea. I can't take out an appendix with this kit, but I can treat the whole range of minor illness and injuries that are likely to crop up on a cruise, and stabilize shipmates with serious illnesses and injuries. I suggest that you buy the items described below that are appropriate to your needs, the medical skills of the best-trained individual on board, and the anticipated length of your voyage. Store them in a readily accessible place on your boat in a large tackle box so that you can easily transfer the kit into a survival craft if you need to abandon ship. And inventory its contents periodically and replace used items and dated medications.

WOUND-CARE MATERIALS

bar soap
antiseptic solution, two 4-oz. bottles
1% silver sulfadiazine cream (Silvadene), 400-gram jar
bulb irrigating syringe, 60 cc
two 20-cc syringes with 20 gauge needles
antibiotic ointment, two 1-oz tubes (Neosporin, Bacitracin)
15 Adaptic dressings, 3" x 3"
24 sterile dressing pads, 4" x 4"
10 Kerlix or Kling roll bandages, 4" x 5 yds
8 Surgipads, 8" x 10", or ABD pads, 8" x 8"
2 rolls waterproof adhesive tape, 1" x 5 yds
8 Bioclusive or Tegaderm transparent dressings, 2" x 3" or
  3" x 3"
Spenco 2nd Skin
surgical staples (Precise Five-shot, 3M)
50 bandage strips (Band-Aids), 1" x 3"
20 skin-closure strips, 1/4" x 3"
20 skin-closure strips, 1/2" x 3"
compound benzoin tincture, 2 oz.
4 sterile eye pads
2 metal eye shields
Q-tip cotton swabs
silver nitrate sticks
[Store dressings and bandages in plastic bags or a water-tight
  plastic container.]

Bar soap. Use to clean abrasions and superficial cuts and burns.
Antiseptic solution. Chlorhexidine (Hibiclens), Povidone-iodine
  (Betadine), and benzalkonium chloride are powerful germi-
  cides that should be used to clean open wounds.
Silver sulfadiazine cream is a topical antimicrobial used on burns
  to prevent infection.
Bulb irrigating syringe can be used to irrigate wounds or to flush
  foreign matter from the eyes.

Syringes and needles are for irrigating wounds.

Antibiotic ointment. Dab a little on abrasions and cuts before applying a dressing. It's good for facial burns, too.

Adaptic pads. These nonadherent pads can be applied directly to a wound and won't stick.

Sterile dressing pads. Use them to clean or dress wounds. Their wicking action absorbs blood and fluids.

Kling and Kerlix bandages. These stretchy gauze rolls are terrific for securing splints, or as the final layer in a bulky wound dressing.

Surgipads/ABDs are ideal for applying pressure to bleeding wounds and as burn coverings.

Bioclusive or Tegaderm dressings are transparent dressings that keep out water and dirt, but not air. You can apply them to small cuts, abrasions, and blisters.

Spenco 2nd Skin is a hydrogel that makes a soothing dressing for open blisters and burns.

Skin closure strips. Take your pick from Steri-Strips (3M), Butterflies (Johnson & Johnson), Coverstrip Closures (Beiersdorf), or Curi-Strips (Kendall). These easy-to-apply paper strips can be used to close most small lacerations. They'll stick better if you apply *tincture of benzoin* to the wound edges first.

Silver nitrate sticks are used to cauterize nosebleeds.

MEDICATIONS

100 analgesic tablets (aspirin, acetaminophen, or ibuprofen)
60 dimenhydrinate (Dramamine) 50-mg tablets, or 20 meclizine (Antivert) 25-mg tablets
*12 Transderm Scōp patches
30 diphenhydramine (Benadryl) 25-mg tabs
Donnagel, 4 oz
30 Imodium tablets
*10 Phenergan (promethazine) 25-mg rectal suppositories

*30 Tylenol No. 3 tablets
*30 Vicodin ES tablets
*Nubain 10 mg/cc, 10-cc multi-use vial (injectable narcotic
    analgesic for severe pain)
*30 triazolam (Halcion) 0.25-mg tablets
*100 penicillin VK 250-mg tablets
*100 trimethoprim-sulfamethoxazole [TMP-SMX] (Bactrim
    DS) 800/160-mg tablets
*100 tetracycline 500-mg tablets
*20 ciprofloxacin (Cipro) 500-mg tablets
*100 amoxicillin (Amoxil) 250-mg tablets
*20 cefadroxil (Duricef) 500-mg tablets
Maalox or Mylanta, 20 oz
Caladryl lotion, 8 oz
12 Domeboro tablets
500 Vitamin C 50-mg tablets
*sulfacetamide 10% ophthalmic drops, 10 cc
tetrahydrozoline eye drops, 0.05%, ½ oz (Visine)
*2% homatropine eye drops, 1 oz
*tetracaine ophthalmic drops, 1 oz
Lotrimin cream 1%, 30 g
hydrocortisone 1% cream, 2 oz
*30 prednisone 20-mg tablets
Solarcaine first-aid lotion, 3 oz
sunscreen SPF 15 or greater, several bottles
zinc oxide, 2 oz
Cavit, 7-gram tube
Desitin ointment
5 one-liter bags of Ringer's lactate intravenous solution
Intravenous tubing; intravenous catheters, 16 and 18 gauge,
    5 of each
Isopropyl alcohol
Milk of magnesia
Eucerin with PABA
Personal medications
*Prescription medicines. Show this list to your physician. He
    can tailor it to your particular medical needs.

Dramamine, meclizine and *Transderm Scōp* patches are sea-sickness remedies.

Diphenhydramine (Benadryl) is an antihistamine used to treat allergic reactions, itching, nausea, and insomnia.

Donnagel is liquid gold when diarrhea strikes. Keep some *Imodium* tablets in the kit in case the Donnagel doesn't do the job.

Phenergan suppositories control vomiting and seasickness.

Tylenol No. 3. Each tablet contains 300 mg of acetaminophen and 30 mg of codeine. It relieves moderately severe pain, cough, and diarrhea.

Vicodin ES tablets contain the narcotic hydrocodone, 7.5 mg, and acetaminophen, 750 mg. Save these for moderately severe pain that doesn't respond to Tylenol No. 3.

Nubain is a potent narcotic analgesic. Inject 10 mg into the shoulder muscle (deltoid) every 3 to 6 hours for severe pain.

Triazolam is a safe, reliable sleeping tablet.

Trimethoprim-sulfamethoxazole, tetracycline, cefadroxil, amoxicillin, penicillin VK, and *ciprofloxacin* are antibiotics.

Caladryl dries and takes the itch out of poison ivy rashes.

Domeboro tablets can be used to make Burow's solution, an astringent, drying solution for poison ivy rash.

Vitamin C tablets will prevent scurvy, a potential problem for castaways.

Tetrahydrozoline drops (Visine a.c.) soothe smoke- or sun-reddened eyes.

2% Homatropine drops dilate the pupil and relieve the pain of corneal abrasions and traumatic iritis.

Sulfacetamide ophthalmic drops are used to treat bacterial eye infections.

Tetracaine drops are used to anesthetize the cornea so as to allow a thorough exam. (WARNING! Repeat dosing with tetracaine retards healing of corneal injuries and predisposes the eye to additional trauma.)

Lotrimin cream kills athlete's foot, jock itch, and vaginal fungi.

Prednisone is a powerful anti-inflammatory steroid.

Cavit is a dental paste for emergency dental repairs.

Zinc oxide is a physical sunblock.

Desitin ointment helps to heal skin fissures, cracks, and ulcers.

Isopropyl alcohol, in a 40 to 70% solution, can be used to in-activate coelenterate venom.

Milk of magnesia is an old standby for constipation.

Eucerin with PABA is a great moisturing lotion for dry skin and salt sores.

MISCELLANEOUS

4 rubberized (ACE) bandages, 3″ and 6″
4 instant cold packs
bee-sting allergy kit (Ana-Kit)
cravats
30 large safety pins
12 tongue blades
tweezers
hemostats, 2 straight and 2 curved
No. 3 stainless steel scalpel handle
Nos. 10, 11, and 20 scalpel blades, 3 of each
scissors
single-edge razor
pliers
moleskin
thermometer
pen light
Sawyer Extractor
magnifying glass
SAM splint
air splint
aluminum splint
wire splint
enema kit
splinter forceps
blood pressure cuff
stethoscope
water-purification tablets (Potable Aqua, Globuline, Hala-zone)
A compendium of your medical history (including family and

personal history, operations, immunizations, allergies, list of prescription medications, a copy of your latest EKG, and names and phone numbers of physicians) A copy of this book and the Merck Manual

Rubberized bandages are indispensable for wrapping sprains, securing splints to fractured limbs, and applying compression dressings to bruised muscles and large wounds.

An **insect sting kit** (Ana-Kit) containing antihistamine tablets and a syringe loaded with adrenaline is essential if you or any of your shipmates has a history of severe insect sting reactions. Available by prescription.

A **cravat** is a triangular muslin bandage that you can use to make a sling or turban bandage, or to secure splints to fractured limbs.

Safety pins can be used to hold your glasses together if you lose a screw, keep the airway open in an unconscious person, close gaping wounds, drain blisters and abscesses, remove splinters, and secure bandages, splints, and slings.

Tongue blades are ideal for applying ointment to abrasions, rashes, or burns, and make good splints for fractured or dislocated fingers.

Needle-nose pliers are handy for removing fishhooks.

Moleskin can be applied over blisters.

The **Sawyer Extractor** is useful for removing venom from wasp and bee stings and venomous fish wounds.

The **SAM splint** is a versatile light, padded, malleable splint for fractured limbs.

Air splints are comfortable and easy to apply.

An **enema kit** may be one of your most treasured items on a long offshore cruise.

The **Merck Manual** is a medical compendium that covers every disease, from asthma to yaws. It's available at most bookstores.

CAVEAT: Readers with chronic medical problems or a history of drug allergy, as well as all pregnant or breast-feeding women, should consult their physicians before taking any of the medications recommended in this book.

INDEX

Page numbers in *italics* refer to illustrations.

ABOUT THE AUTHOR

Paul G. Gill, Jr., grew up in Stony Brook, New York, where he first developed his love for boating and the sea. He attended the University of Notre Dame and the University of Alabama School of Medicine, and now practices emergency medicine in Vermont. He writes a sports medicine column for *Outdoor Life* magazine, and spends much of his leisure time sailing or motorboating on Lake Champlain and Lake George. His first book, *Simon & Schuster's Pocket Guide to Wilderness Medicine*, was published in 1991.